D1561121

Vagus Nerve

The Survival Guide to Vagus Nerve
Healing, Self Hypnosis, Cognitive
Behavioral Therapy, Empath Healing and
Anger Management for Overcome Anxiety,
Depression, Trauma and Stop Hidden
Abuse

Dr. Stanley Leary

Legal & Disclaimer

The information contained in this book and its contents is not designed to replace or take the place of any form of medical or professional advice; and is not meant to replace the need for independent medical, financial, legal or other professional advice or services, as may be required. The content and information in this book has been provided for educational and entertainment purposes only.

The content and information contained in this book has been compiled from sources deemed reliable, and it is accurate to the best of the Author's knowledge, information and belief. However, the Author cannot guarantee its accuracy and validity and cannot be held liable for any errors and/or omissions. Further, changes are periodically made to this book as and when needed. Where appropriate and/or necessary, you must consult a professional (including but not limited to your doctor, attorney, financial advisor or such other professional advisor) before using any of the suggested remedies, techniques, or information in this book.

Upon using the contents and information contained in this book, you agree to hold harmless the Author from and against any damages, costs, and expenses, including any legal fees potentially resulting from the application of any of the information provided by this book. This disclaimer applies to any loss, damages or injury caused by the use and application, whether directly or indirectly, of any advice or information presented, whether for breach of

Table of Contents

INTRODUCTION

The vagus nerve is called as a vagabond, which sends sensory fibers to visceral organs from the brain stem. The vagus nerve, the longest of the cranial nerves, configures your nerve center the parasympathetic system.

And it controls a wide range of critical features, which transmit sensory impulses and engines to each organ in your body.

Recent studies have shown that the connection to the management of chronic inflammation and the start of an exciting new field of therapy for serious, incurable diseases may also be missing.

Let me share nine facts about this powerful nerve bundle.

A Virginia Faculty study of rats showed that the stimulation of their vagus nerves strengthened their memories.

The activity presented the norepinephrine neurotransmitter to the amygdala that consolidated memories.

Similar research trials in humans have been completed, indicating possible approaches to Alzheimer's disease issues.

The vagus nerve neurotransmitter acetylcholine directs your lungs to breathe.

It has a major reason why Botox is often used cosmetically because it interrupts your production of acetylcholine. Nevertheless, your vagus nerve can definitely be stimulated with abdominal breathing or with your breath held for 4 to 8 counts.

Vagus is a visceral motor for all endothoracic organs (pharynx, larynx, esophagus, heart, lungs) and for many subdiaphragmatic organs (surreni, kidneys, stomach, first half of the large intestine).

The vagus nerve, the primary patron of the parasympathetic sensory system, is the tenth cranial nerve beginning from the medulla oblongata in the focal sensory system. Inside the medulla, the cell groups of vagal preganglionic neurons are found in the core uncertain (NA) and the dorsal engine of the vagus (DMV). These cores supply fibres to the vagus nerve, which rises up out of the head by means of the jugular foramen.

At the degree of the jugular foramen, the unrivaled jugular ganglion of the vagus gives cutaneous branches to the auriculus and outside acoustic meatus. Only distally, there is a subsequent ganglion, alluded to as the no dose ganglion, gathering tactile innervation from instinctive organs. The cell assortments of follower (for example tactile) neurons are situated in the last ganglion and undertaking to the core of the singular tract (NTS). This core transfers contribution to the medulla so as to manage the cardiovascular, respiratory and gastrointestinal (GI) functions. The cervical vagus plunges inside the carotid sheath close by the carotid supply route and interior jugular vein. Cardiovascular vagal branches leave the cervical vagus and join the heart plexus.

The left and right intermittent laryngeal nerve, emerging at the degree of the aortic curve and subclavian supply route individually, additionally add to the cardiovascular innervation. Other than the heart, the two vagi innervate the lungs through the pneumonic plexus vagus, separately. Notwithstanding, one needs to remember that every trunk gets fibres from both cervical vagus nerves. The quantity of back and foremost trunks going through the diaphragmatic opening is variable, up to two in the previous and three in the last mentioned. The front trunk disseminates gastric branches to the foremost part of the stomach and gives of a hepatic branch. Other than innervating the liver, the hepatic stem gives of branches to the pylorus and the proximal piece of the duodenum and pancreas. Then again, the back trunk disseminates one gastric

7

branch to the proximal back part of the stomach and another to the coeliac plexus, which innervates the spleen and GI tract coming to the extent the left colonic flexure. The internal organ gets extra parasympathetic innervation through the pelvic splanchnic nerve (S2-S4), which ends in the pelvic plexus and develops as the colonic and rectal nerve.

The follower vagus nerve innervates the GI tract by means of vagal terminals both in the lamina propria and in the muscularis externa. In any case, the edherent vagus nerve fibres just cooperate with neurons of the enteric sensory system (ENS). The ENS comprises out of a thick meshwork of nerve fibres, arranged in the submucosal (for example submucosal plexus) and outside strong compartment of the digestive system (for example myenteric plexus). By methods for electrophysiological and anterograde tracer ponders, it was shown that preganglionic parasympathetic fibres (for example both vagal and sacral innervation) legitimately interface with different postganglionic myenteric neurons by development of varicosities, though couple of vagal fibres speak with submucosal neurons.

The preganglionic innervation of the GI tract shows a run of the mill rostro-caudal angle with the most noteworthy thickness of innervated myenteric neurons in the stomach and duodenum pursued by a dynamic decrease in the small digestive system and colon. The way that gastric myenteric neurons are initiated by vagal information was likewise shown immunohistochemically with the recognition of c-Fos and phosphorylated c-AMP reaction component restricting protein (p-CREB), which are markers for neuronal action. As actuation of neurons inside one ganglion is started after a similar inactivity period, Schemann et al. propose that the vagal contribution to the ENS is single reflex. Be that as it may, this isn't confirmed by different investigations. Right now, three unmistakable vagal follower terminals have been portrayed. The specific area of every terminal has relationships with its physiological capacity.

Part 1: The Science

Chapter 1: What is Vagus Nerve

As a treatment target of gastrointestinal and psychiatric disorders such as inflammatory bowel disease (IBD), anxiety, and post-traumatic stress disorder (PTSD), the brain-good axis is becoming increasingly important. The gut is an essential immune system control center and the immune modulator property of the vagus nerve.

As a consequence, this nerve plays a significant role in the gut, heart, and inflammatory relationship. For starters, vagus nerve stimulation (VNS), or meditation techniques, there are new treatment approaches to modulate the brain–good axis. For mood and anxiety problems, but also in other conditions associated with increased inflammation, these therapies are effective. Gut-directed hypnotherapy is especially effective in both irritable bowel syndrome and IBD.

Extensive evidence is also available in treatment-resistant depression for the application of invasive VNS therapy. Small studies and case study series have shown the efficacy of intrusive VNS in treating refractory migraine and cluster headache, Alzheimer's disease, anxiety disorders resistant to medication, bipolar disorder, and obesity. To improve efficacy and safety, numerous VNS instruments have been developed over the years. We will discuss the latest advances in invasive VNS technology for the treatment of epilepsy, more recently developed invasive VNS devices for other uses than systems for epilepsy and anxiety, and non-invasive vagus nerve stimulation.

The vagus nerve is the major aspect of the parasympathetic nervous system, which controls a wide range of vital body functions, including attitude regulation, immune response, metabolism, and heart rate. There is preliminary evidence that activation of the vagus nerve is a promising potential therapy for medication-refractory anxiety, posttraumatic stress disorder and inflammatory disease of the intestine.

Chapter 2: Where is the Vagus Nerve located

Here's what we are experiencing every day: after eating, we feel tired. This is like a slight drowsiness that encourages you to sit on the couch and relax or take a short nap.

This sensation is regulated by the vagus nerve. After eating, our bodies consume a lot of energy to do digestion.

Therefore, this nerve triggers a series of stimuli to promote calmness and classic "sleepiness".

In addition to controlling digestion, the vagus nerve monitors that the heart is not overexcited. Therefore, the vagus nerve causes loss of consciousness. Those are extreme cases.

It also regulates the immune system and cell regeneration. On the other hand, another feature of this attractive structure is to give you a feeling of fullness.

Since it is closely related to the digestive process, it also functions as a regulator.

This tells us that we already have enough, and when we suffer from stress, he tells us that we have more cravings or less appetite.

As you can see, it is a natural complement in various fields, such as relaxation, fullness, weight, and more or less anxiety.

The vagus nerve likewise called pneumogastric nerve, cranial nerve X, the Wanderer or now and then the Rambler, is the tenth of twelve (barring CN0) combined cranial nerves. Other than yield to the different organs in the body the vagus nerve passes on tangible data about the condition of the body's organs to the focal sensory system. 80-90% of the nerve filaments in the vagus nerve are afferent (tactile) nerves imparting the condition of the viscera to the mind.

The medieval Latin word vagus implies actually "Meandering" (the words transient, drifter, and obscure originate from a similar root).

Innervation

Both right and left vagus nerves plummet from the cerebrum in the carotid sheath, horizontal to the carotid corridor.

The correct vagus nerve offers ascend to the privilege repetitive laryngeal nerve which snares around the privilege subclavian vein and rises into the neck between the trachea and throat. The correct vagus at that point crosses anteriorly to the privilege subclavian corridor and runs back to the better vena cava and drops back than the correct principle bronchus and adds to heart, pneumonic and esophageal plexuses. It shapes the back vagal trunk at the lower some portion of the throat and enters the stomach through the esophageal break.

The left vagus further radiates thoracic cardiovascular branches, separates into aspiratory plexus, proceeds into the esophageal plexus and enters the guts as the front vagal trunk in the esophageal break of the stomach.

The vagus nerve supplies engine parasympathetic filaments to every one of the organs with the exception of the suprarenal (adrenal) organs, starting from the neck to the second fragment of the transverse colon.

This implies the vagus nerve is liable for such fluctuated assignments as pulse, gastrointestinal peristalsis, perspiring, and many muscle developments in the mouth, including discourse (through the repetitive laryngeal nerve) and keeping the larynx open for breathing (by means of activity of the back cricoarytenoid muscle, the main abductor of the vocal folds). It additionally has some afferent strands that innervate the internal (channel) bit of the

14

external ear, by means of the Auricular branch (otherwise called Alderman's nerve) and part of the meninges. This clarifies why an individual may hack when tickled on their ear, (for example, when attempting to expel ear wax with a cotton swab).

Chapter 3: Functions of the Vagus Nerve

The vagus nerve links the brainstem on the entire body. It enables the brain to monitor as well as receive info about a number of the body's various functions.

You will find two separate central nervous system capabilities offered by the vagus nerve and its related parts.

The nerve is liable for some sensory-motor and activity info for action in the entire body.

Basically, it's an element of a circuit that links the neck, lungs, heart, and the abdomen on the human brain.

The vagus nerve has a variety of functions. The four crucial features of the vagus nerve are:

Sensory: From the throat, lungs, heart, and belly.

Exclusive sensory: Provides taste sensation behind the tongue.

Motor: Provides action operates for all the muscles in the neck accountable for swallowing and speech.

Parasympathetic: Accountable for the intestinal tract, heart rate functioning, and respiration.

Its functions of its could be broken down even more into seven categories.

One of those is controlling the central nervous system.

The central nervous system may be split into two areas: parasympathetic and sympathetic.

The sympathetic side increases alertness, heart rate, blood pressure, energy, and breathing rate.

The parasympathetic side that the vagus nerve is highly involved in decreases alertness, blood pressure, and pulse rate, and also will help with calmness, rest, and break down of food.

As an outcome, the vagus nerve likewise helps with sexual arousal, urination, and defecation.

Some other vagus nerve consequences include Communication between the gut and the brain: The vagus nerve provides info from the gut on the human brain.

Leisure with serious breathing: The vagus nerve sends a message to the diaphragm. Along with deep breaths, an individual feels much more relaxed.

Lowering inflammation: The vagus nerve also sends a signal to various other areas of the body in the form of an anti-inflammatory signal.

Decreasing the blood pressure and heart rate:

This was regarded as a genuine state of the art in precisely how vagus nerve stimulation may not just deal with rheumatoid arthritis but any other inflammatory diseases, like Crohn's, Parkinson's, and Alzheimer's.

To understand the connection between the vagus nerve and depression, we need to realize that the central nervous system consists of two opposing mechanisms that continuously send information on the human brain.

The sympathetic nervous system prepares us for action and feeds stress hormones, mainly as cortisol and adrenaline.

The parasympathetic nervous system intervenes in relaxation.

These approaches serve as decelerators and accelerators in practice.

The sympathetic nervous system strengthens and activates us as the parasympathetic nervous system helps us relax and reduce speed, and neurotransmitters such as acetylcholine decrease the heart rate and blood pressure and make sure the body operates more efficiently.

The features of the vagus nerve regulate the parasympathetic system.

This interferes with various features from mouth to pulse and can lead to different symptoms when affected.

Many of the vagus nerves in our corps are: they help to control the rhythm, monitor the movements of muscle mass, and sustain breathing rate.

It maintains the performance of the intestinal tract and enables food to be processed by contraction of the intestinal and stomach muscles.

It makes it easier to relax after a tense situation, or it means that we are at risk and do not have to lower the guard.

Give sensory information about organ status to the brain.

If stressful conditions are met, the sympathetic nervous system is triggered.

In case the pressure continues, and the physiological reaction that causes it cannot be turned off, it will not take time to face problems.

For mind quantity, two pathways are needed: the hypothalamus-hypophysis-adrenal axis and the axis of the brain intestine.

The brain reacts to pressure and anxiety by rising hormone production (CRF) which travels out of the hypothalamus in the hypophysis gland in which they induce the release of other hormones (ACTH), that travels through the blood to the adrenal gland to facilitate the activation of cortisol and adrenaline, and which is an immune suppressor and an inflammatory precursor of the body;

That's why we're sick readily when we feel pressured and anxious and eventually get depressed, a disorder linked to an inflammatory mental effect.

And chronic anxiety and stress were not enough to produce a higher level of glutamate in the human brain, a neurotransmitter that causes anxiety, depression, and migraine when made extra.

In fact, a great deal of cortisol inhibits the hippocampus, a part of the human brain that is responsible for developing new memories.

Vagus nerve involvement can lead to problems such as dizziness, gastrointestinal problems, arrhythmias, breathing difficulties, and unproportionate emotional reactions.

The vagus nerve cannot activate the leisure signal, and therefore the sympathetic nervous system is active, causing the person to respond impulsively and suffer from anxiety.

In addition, research conducted at the Faculty of Miami has found that the vaguely overall tonic is passed from mother to child.

Women with anxiety, depression, and extreme frustration had a decreased vagal activity during their pregnancy, and their babies had weak vagal activity and lower amounts of serotonin and dopamine.

How often do you experience depression in your daily life?

This section is ideal for you if you are worried about too much or are caught in irrational feelings or being nausea, chest pain, and heart palpitations.

Through stimulating your vagus nerve, you plan to learn a simple but extremely effective technique to cope with anxiety naturally.

This unique and powerful approach can be used at any time and anywhere to relieve anxiety and stress, from home and on the way, and even at all those terrible business meetings.

Have you understood that the FDA approved an operated device to deal with depression effectively by periodically revitalizing the vagus nerve?

Yet you won't need surgery, preferably.

Through performing a variety of simple breathing techniques, you can take advantage of vagus nerve stimulation.

The vagus nerve is the central element of the parasympathetic nervous system (which calms you by controlling your relief).

It comes from your brain and "wanders" into the abdomen through the length of the brains, scattering fibers on your mouth, pharynx, vocal chords, lung, heart, intestines and glands that make anti-stress enzymes and hormones (such as acetylcholine, oxytocin), vasopressin, prolactin, metabolism, and of course the response to relaxation.

Vagus nerve acts as a mind-body connection and is the cable that drives the sensations and intestinal instincts of your brain.

The secret to controlling the mind and anxiety levels lies in their ability to stimulate the parasympathetic system's relaxing nerve pathways.

You cannot manage this specific component of the central nervous system upon request, but you can indirectly promote your vagus nerve by immersing your face in cold waters (diving mirror).

This is often achieved by shutting the eyes or pinching the nose when trying to respire. It dramatically increases stress in the tumor cavity to revitalize the vagus nervousness and improve the vagus voice.

And, obviously, diaphragmic breathing approaches Strengthening it living central nervous system will pay good dividends, and the best way to achieve this by teaching the breath.

Respire with Your Diaphragm

Now it is time to implement this theory. The first thing you need to do is breathe with the diaphragm (abdominal respiration).

This is the basis of proper respiration and stress relief.

The diaphragm is the main muscle of the body.

It's shaped belled, and when you eat it, it's patterns and acts as a piston and produces vacuum in your chest cavity, so your lungs can rise, and the air gets into it.

This causes pressure, on the other hand, pressing down and out the viscera, raising the belly.

That is why good breathing is called abdominal breathing.

Respire with the partially closed glottis Glottis is in the back of your tongue and is shut while you catch a breath.

We want to get it partially closed here. It is the sensation that you get in your throat when you exhale and make a Hhhh noise to purify the lenses, but without actually making the sound.

It also looks like your tactic when you are on the edge of relaxation, and you expect to snore a little.

You control the glottis: Control the airflow during inhalation and exhalation.

Stimulates the Nerve of the Vagus

Now, it is time to apply this whole concept with this seven-eleven diaphragm breathing technique.

Inhale via the nose, with the glottis partially shut down, for example, almost create Hhhh audio for the seven hold breath for a while.

Exhale through the nose (or the mouth), with the glottis partially shut down, such as almost creating HHhh audio for one number of eleven.

The more you practice, the more effective this particular method becomes.

In the end, if your newly acquired breathing skills are created and abdominal breathing becomes a pattern, the body continues to run at a considerably lower stress level.

You will also see (or sometimes you won't) that your breath responds to traumatic situations.

Your body can regulate your breath automatically and, therefore, your anxiety and stress.

One of the ways to deal with fear is how to stimulate the vagus nerve by proper respiration.

The vagus nerve acts as the interface between the mind and the body to regulate the reaction to relaxation.

You can stimulate the vagus nerve with the glottis partially shut.

Use your old days to master this technique, turn it into a routine frequently, and the results shock you.

When you say stress, you're on the right path.

More specifically, they are each due to a lack of vagus activity. But no, not that kind of Vegas.

This particular type of vagus is important to your health and well-being.

In this specific chapter, you will find out why your vagus nerve is very important and how it can calm your nerves, sleep, break down, and promote the natural healing powers of your body.

Your vagus nerve binds your brain to your intestine and your internal organs to the heart.

His effect is so widespread that it is known as "the captain" for your parasympathetic nervous system: the normal stimulation, regeneration, and recovery of the reaction unit of your body.

The adequate output of your vagus nerve keeps chronic inflammation stable, splitting virtually all major diseases.

It controls heart rhythm and maximizes pulse rate variability, which is an important indicator of cardiac health.

And it shows that the lungs breathe deeply, so absorb the oxygen that fills up the vital energy.

Besides, the vagus nerve transfers information from the intestine into the brain that offers intestinal intuition about what's harmful or beneficial to you.

Next, it allows you to consolidate memories, so you remember important information and good intentions.

Eventually, your vagus nerve releases acetylcholine, which helps combat the stress adrenaline and cortisol and activates your body's natural calming response to calm, rest, and heal.

Now you have a PICTURE of why it is so crucial to activate your vagus nerve.

The problem is that our culture today allows us to get extremely busy, very hyper stressed, so that we work in pressure mode almost always, without knowing it.

We are used to the stimulation. We don't know how true relaxation feels, much less how.

We are hyperactive instead of following an all-natural rhythm of rest and action.

And we are so trained that we feel responsible if we don't do something, or if we are not excited yet entertained!

As a consequence, irritability, anxiety, and insomnia are lifelong companions.

It keeps us from sleeping well and leads us to chronic diseases such as cancer.

So how can we break this deadly pattern?

Luckily, the body is very resilient. It's just waiting for you to trigger your organic equilibrium, which is similar to several long, deep breaths.

When you inhale deeply and gradually, you activate your vagus nerve.

It sends soothing signals to lower your brainwave and heart rate and activates all the rest and repair mechanisms of the natural relaxation response of your body.

Slow deep breathing is, therefore, extremely important. Nonetheless, there is a question. Living in continuous stress mode facilitates a restrained, quick, shallow breathing style. Slow deep breathing also usually takes some exercise.

This is a fantastic way to do this: a simple Deep Breathing Meditation: lie on your back and close your eyes carefully.

Rest your hands on your lower abdomen, one and the other.

When you inhale, cause your lower abdomen to ascend as it breathes slowly.

Allow your lower abdomen to relax as you exhale, as it empties.

Sit in a nice, clear rhythm as the abdomen rises and falls gently, following your breath.

Figure out if you cannot stress this but only understand how it happens naturally, quickly.

When you start, make sure you remember the second you begin to inhale and stick to it until you pause.

First, note the second you're beginning to exhale and hold it until you quit.

Follow this soothing rhythm for a few minutes, and then remember how happy you are. Be sure to shoot this at this stage, when you can, so you have it for yourself.

Every day, you can do this simple deep respiratory relaxation to relieve the pressure of the layers and the stress that has taken place from the past. In the night before rest, you can make it lying in bed, to prepare your body to sleep.

Quickly in all, you reset the internal balance of your body, resulting in a much safer, happier, and peaceful life.

Chapter 4: How the Vagus Nerve manages it all.

The vagus nerve manages so many parts of the body that it can be devastating when something goes wrong. If there is anything that damages the nerve, such as medication, trauma, or disease, can the body heal itself? Or are you stuck with nerve damage for the rest of your life? It really all depends on how bad the damage is. Nerve damage is notorious for being slow to heal and the vagus nerve is no exception. However, scientists have tested the ability of the vagus nerve to regenerate in rats and the results have been surprising. Not only have vagus nerve techniques helped with the restoration of the central vagal parts, but they have also been shown to increase synaptic plasticity. This means that even when the brain suffers damage from damage done to the vagus nerve, it can be reversed, to a certain extent.

In tests done on rats, it took roughly 4.5 months to regenerate the central vagal nerve. That's good news for people, though it hasn't been fully tested in humans. However, studies have also shown that rebuilding the nerves in the gastrointestinal tract did not occur over the course of 45 weeks, or almost a year, which is how long the study lasted. It will definitely take time for nerves to grow back and regenerate, but the fact that it is actually possible could be exactly the hope we need.

While the central sections of the vagal nerve can be regenerated surprisingly quickly, it takes much longer to regrow the areas that branch out from it. It's important to note this because you shouldn't expect instant results from the exercises and techniques given in this book. It takes time to heal nerve damage, and that means you need to be patient and consistent if you have suffered from vagal nerve damage. Stimulation of the vagus nerve can help it grow and recover from damage. Again, it takes time, but if you are willing to put in the time and effort, you'll find that things gradually get better. As many people have discovered before you, this is not a trick. Vagus nerve stimulation really works and it can have an incredible impact on your life.

I went from barely being able to move around my house, to running marathons again. I've seen other people do even more miraculous things. And it really does seem like a miracle, but it's actually just science and your nervous system, doing their jobs. With the right stimulation, your vagus nerve will start working better than ever and becomes even more efficient. Even if you haven't suffered from any particular trauma or nerve damage, you can still expect some results from toning up your vagus nerve. It can only help you feel better and ensure that your body runs more efficiently. The amount of energy you'll have will increase and you will find that it is easier to live the lifestyle you want. There's an amazing amount of information out there if you know what to look for, yet it's still not common knowledge. I find this flabbergasting, but here you'll learn everything you need to know about how to stimulate your vagus nerve and help it recover.

Part 2: What could go wrong in Vagus?

Chapter 5: Dysfunctional Breathing

The Vagus nerve has the primary function of offering stimulation to the vocal chord's muscles. If your vagus nerve has any sort of damage or dysfunction, there is a probability that these muscles will be damaged as well. This then interferes with both your breathing ability and your voice. Other muscles are supported by the function of the Vagus nerve as well. You may feel like your electrolytes are low, such as your potassium or magnesium levels, which cause muscle cramps, but those cramps may also be caused by damage to your Vagus nerve.

Poor circulation: In some people, poor circulation is an unpleasant sign of a low vagal tone. When your hands and feet tend to get cold, but the rest of the body is fine, it may be caused by a lack of circulation. The blood just isn't reaching as far as it should. Since the vagus nerve is responsible for your heart rate, it is a big part of this disease and needs to be considered when dealing with low circulation.

Pulmonary disease: Your lungs are also controlled by the vagus nerve and it stimulates regular breathing. Poor lung health, COPD, and other types of pulmonary disease can all affect the vagal tone in the body.

When you are frightened, have you ever noticed how your breathing picks up? This is in response to your sympathetic nervous system— your body is literally being pushed into fight-flight-freeze mode in preparation to keep itself alive. When you wish to calm yourself down from those feelings of panic, you may unconsciously put yourself through deep breathing exercises in an attempt to regulate yourself. Do you know why?

Most people do not realize it, but those deep breaths actually are triggering to your vagus nerve that it is time to get to work. The vagus nerve is essentially goaded into acting in a way that will allow for the alleviation of symptoms and slowing of the heart rate because the vagus nerve activates the parasympathetic nervous system.

Without the vagus nerve and this little feedback loop, your heart rate would likely sit around 100 bpm naturally. It would rarely drop lower, and your heart rate would be free to skyrocket without limitation, which of course, could be dangerous. The parasympathetic nervous system keeps that from happening— the parasympathetic system's purpose is essentially to put the brakes on the sympathetic nervous system. It is the regulator— the part of you that is able to calm you down and convince you to relax. It slows your heart rate and helps you achieve that state of calm that you may be looking for after an anxiety attack.

When you are breathing, have you ever noticed how your heart rate changes? When you take in a deep breath, you may feel your pulse quicken, and as you exhale, you notice it drop again. This is for a very specific reason— your vagus nerve is regulating your heart rate. When you breathe in, you trigger your pulse to quicken, and as your pulse quickens, it raises blood pressure.

That raise in blood pressure and pulse triggers your parasympathetic nervous system to kick in— it wants to regulate your heart rate, so it dumps some acetylcholine into your blood stream, slowing the heart rate. This is important to keep in mind— it means that you can effectively kick your vagus nerve into action simply by taking a deep breath in and cuing to the nerve that you are in need of some regulation to keep your heart rate steady. Your vagus nerve, as you exhale, is at its most active, slowing your heart rate the most. This means, then, that you are able to effectively regulate yourself and your parasympathetic nervous system all through breathing.

This is nothing new— in fact, the breathing pattern that triggers this state of calmness thanks to the parasympathetic nervous system actually arises in several different calming, spiritual activities. Mantras used during any sort of meditation can trigger this sort of activation, creating the proper timing between breaths and holding them, as do saying the Ave Maria prayer. The breathing rate during these techniques is dropped down to about six breaths every minute, which is what these breathing techniques will aim for.

Chapter 6: Dysfunctional Digestive Sequence

When the vagus nerve is damaged or malfunctioning, it can affect the digestive system; a condition known as digestive gastroparesis occurs when the muscles in the stomach are unable to process and move food forward to the small intestine. Peristalsis, the contracts and expansions that advance the food do not function effectively.

The causes of digestive gastroparesis are often unknown but in addition to a damaged vagus nerve (caused by surgery, for example), it may be caused by uncontrolled diabetes, narcotics and medications, Parkinson's disease, multiple sclerosis, and in very rare cases, certain connective tissue disorders.

Symptoms range from heartburn and GERD (acid reflux complications), bloating, loss of appetite and feeling full prematurely, and nausea. Undigested food that remains in the stomach may ferment and be susceptible to bacterial infection.

Here is what is essential to understand: health is accomplished when the body is capable of protecting itself from imbalances, collapse, and foreign invaders. The human body has developed potent protection systems to maintain optimum mental, physical and emotional conditions. Research shows clear links between our inherent health protection systems and the foods that enable them.

My work allowed me to focus on main body defense systems such as angiogenesis, stem cells, immunity, microbiota, and conservation of DNA. Angiogenesis is the body's mechanism of building new blood vessels. It's the power of our body to keep going.

Stem cells or the capacity of our body to regenerate are essential to the wellbeing of all of our brain tissues and organs, from our hearts to our skin. Immunity is of paramount importance. Everything is about how well our bodies can fight disease and infection. It's all about having a strong immune system.

Our own bacteria are the microbiota. In our body, there are 37 trillion bacteria and we discover that they're not only harmful as we once believed but that they actually help our bodies improve safety.

Health safety for DNA is important. Every day, we have 60,000 mutations in our Genes. Why don't we get cancer more frequently? Okay, our DNA can restore itself - and diet can improve these repair mechanisms.

While Western society has access to the world's most sophisticated drugs, it is sicker than ever. We now live in a culture that promotes "a pill for every illness." One in three of us is expected to be affected by cancer and most of us now know, unfortunately, that at least one person has been affected by a life-changing disease. How sad that humanity is being ravaged by an outbreak of ill health in this era of technical progress.

We were never so disassociated from our bodies and how to regenerate them. They treat illness signs as pain rather than understanding that these symptoms are our way to communicate intelligently with us. Of starters, we can see a headache as an irritation and a paracetamol pop, ignoring the fact that our body let us know it is dehydrated and needs more fluid. Missing these signals means ignoring the warning light or our vehicle dashboard, something that most of us think is highly unwise.

Although the health and healthcare industry is booming recently, many of us do not yet fully appreciate how our lifestyle and dietary choices really impact our well-being. We eat food because its nutritional content and/or its potential to heal is easy or healthy, and very rarely. A heavy intake of gluten, glucose, caffeine, and alcohol is highly toxic, placing the body under immense stress and allowing the virus to flourish under acidic conditions.

The essence of Mother gives us all we need to survive without sickness, and yet surprisingly we preferred low-nutrition pseudo-foods. The body works always to restore balance or homeostasis. The effect is incredible as we learn to work for, not against this inherent intuitive healing. You should predict increased energy, better appetite, loss of weight, better mood and sleep by applying these basic health hacks to your everyday lives.

The natural healing ability of your body is linked to a part of your nervous system known as the autonomous nervous system. It consists of two coordinating components: the sympathetic nervous system and the sympathetic nervous system. The sympathetic system controls the body's "fight or flight" reaction which regulates the relaxing and digesting response in the parasympathetic nervous system.

The nervous system is compassionate to safety when we must avoid risk in brief fires. Now people are constantly anxious and the sympathetic nervous system is stimulated because of no apparent "risk." Once our body feels that it is in danger, our hearts beat harder, our blood flows from lungs and into our bodies to brace us to combat, our analytical thinking, amongst others, will cease. In other words, it actually develops problems for obesity, diabetes, heart disease, and indigestion.

For many medical conditions, it can be detrimental to spend even more in physical treatments and procedures while reducing appointment times and slashing medical staff. One study found that sick patients with irritable bowel syndrome had much significantly greater symptom relief if the doctor was warm and compassionate than cold but polite— irrespective of treatment. Similarly, after prolonged (42-minute) visits with a doctor, patients with acid reflux disease improved dramatically compared to normal (18-minute) appointment. For cases from back pain to pregnancy, the outcomes of patients not only depend on what medications are administered but also on how treatment is taken.

But not all of that. The intelligence does not necessarily assess our subjective experience since the brain regulates bodily processes from metabolism to the immune system; it can be important for the physical progression of the disease as well. Such procedures are not necessarily voluntary; we can't "wish" ourselves more. Nevertheless, we can influence them, particularly by modulating our stress response.

For example, if you are nervous, the heart beats quicker, making the cardiovascular system stronger. This is normally no concern, but it may be dangerous or even deadly in some circumstances. Natural disasters such as earthquakes often kill as many people as they collapse from heart attacks. Studies have shown that people who experience depression or depression beforehand suffer more risks during intrusive medical treatments such as breast biopsies or removal of tumors (for example, lengthy oxygen deficiency, low or high blood pressure, postoperative bleeding or abnormally slow heart rates). Relief strategies such as visualizing a safe location greatly reduce pain and anxiety during these treatments and the risk of adverse events.

Stress can also have physical effects on the intestines. If we are upset with toiletries, we might not go for days, but faced with a task like an interview or a competition will force us to clear our bowels. Such mechanisms worsen problems like IBS and studies indicate that intestinal hypnotherapy which helps clinicians deal with stress and relax their digestive system is highly effective. A course of hypnotherapy decreases intestinal resistance to pain, and while people are hypnotized, they may change their intestinal contractions, something we usually don't do at will.

Third, the body's first line of defense against disease, or trauma, is the division of the immune system called inflammation. This is effective in a crisis, but when caused by chronic stress over the longer term, it interferes with healthy immune responses and eats away the tissues of the skin, leaving us more susceptible to inflammation, allergies, and autoimmune diseases. And not just eczema flare-ups or a couple of extra colds. Stress itself has been shown to increase the development of life-threatening diseases such as multiple sclerosis and HIV through its effects on the immune system. Work that stress-reduction strategies may reverse these changes is only just underway, but some preliminary evidence shows that stress-management counseling can avoid development into MS, and that mindfulness training may delay HIV.

There is even confirmation that the imagination has a role to play in cancer. Inflammation removes damaged cells and facilitates the growth of new blood vessels that are good for healing wounds but that also allows tumors space and nutrients to expand. Stress hormones spread more rapidly in animal studies, while patient studies suggest that stress management interventions decrease inflammation, although the judging panel still examines how much this feeds in improved times of survival.

Even if stress reduction does not directly affect cancer survival, though, behavioral strategies may enhance physiological prognosis in other ways. When chemotherapy relieves fatigue and vomiting which allows someone to stick to their medication schedule, it can improve longevity. Social support, meanwhile, allows patients to make better choices. For one study, patients receiving early palliative care for terminal cancer opted for less aggressive treatment. People were less stressed, better living-and people lived longer.

Mind can not cure anything, and medical therapy is risky and unnecessary in the face of life-threatening circumstances. Yet our mental state has far-ranging physiological effects that can impair health in a wide variety of ways and even in the most serious conditions such as diabetes, multiple sclerosis, and HIV.

Cynics are correct to caution about unfounded findings of psychological physiotherapy. But the rejection of the psychological function has its own dangers. This pushes people - especially those with direct experience in how it can benefit-away from the sciences and to the crackpots of other counselors. And it blinds us to knowledge which might be extremely important for medicine. I argue at Cure that both strategies have to be combined: to provide for the bodies and minds of the patients.

The automatic mode of body healing is triggered when the body is calm and relaxed. The parasympathetic nervous system is in this case dominant. The task of the parasympathetic nervous system is to resist infection in the long run. It regulates your metabolism and other essential processes to stabilize the body.

Did you notice that some individuals regularly get sick while others barely get sick (even when they get sick, they recover fast)?? Those who are "usually" ill are most likely exhausted or distracted -they don't allow their bodies an opportunity to rest and to repair themselves naturally.

Here are the three steps to recover the natural healing mode of your body:

1. Feel Your Body Heat

The temperature of the skin is correlated with the immune system. The ideal body temperature equilibrium is to keep your head cold and warm under the belly. Your lower abdomen is the heart of your body, which encourages wellness by retaining the strength in this area. It's best to increase your body's temperature by having a few minutes ' sunshine or by running to heat your body at least once a day.

2. Control Your Breathing

Practice deep breathing into the diaphragm and lower belly. Deep breathing helps and automatically relieves the skin. While it is very difficult to deliberately increase or decrease blood pressure, heartbeat or body temperature, we will unconsciously regulate it through our breathing. You will also realize that when you concentrate on your breathing, your emotions and thoughts settle and your body is back in balance.

3. Observe With Your Mind

Practice daily mindfulness in a clear and calm mind. Watch your emotions and thoughts and learn not to completely destroy or control them. As you hear the breathing, it deepens and slows down naturally. If you look at the temperature of your skin, it gets safe.

These three actions: sense your body heat, regulate your breathing and watching your mind intertwine in order to create a natural method of preserving the physical health of your body.

Chapter 7: Dysfunctional Microbiome

In the microbiota of one organism, the number of genes in all the bacteria is over 200 times the number of genes in the human genome. The microbiome can weigh up to five pounds.

What does the microbiome have to do with health?

For human development, immunity, and nutrition, the microbiome is essential. Not invaders, but beneficial colonizers are the bacteria that live in and on us. Microbes that cause infection to develop over time, modifying gene expression and metabolic processes, resulting in an unusual immune response to chemicals and tissues that are usually present in the body.

Autoimmune diseases do not seem to be transmitted through inheritance of DNA in families but an inheritance of the microbiome of the body. Few examples: between overweight and slim twins, the gut microbiome is unique. Obese twins have reduced bacterial diversity and higher enzyme rates, which means that obese twins are more effective in digesting food and calorie production. A bad balance of bacteria in the stomach was also associated with obesity.

Type I diabetes is an autoimmune disease related to a less stable intestinal microbiome. Bacteria play an important role in the development of diabetes in animal studies.

Dust from dog homes can reduce the immune response to allergens and other triggers of asthma by changing the gut microbiome composition. Children living in pet homes are shown to be less likely to develop allergies with kids.

What is the Human Microbiome Project (HMP)?

The human microbiome is mapped by worldwide scientific projects, giving insight into uncharted species and genomes. \

Another project, funded by the National Human Genome Research Institute (NHGRI), part of the National Institutes of Health (NIH), is the Human Microbiome Project (HMP). The HMP launched as an extension of the Human Genome Project in 2008. It is a five-year feasibility study with a $ 150 million budget and is being conducted in some centers around the United States.

The HMP aims to research the human being as a supra-organism consisting of non-human and human cells to describe the human microbiome and examine its role in human health and disease.

The HMP's main objective is to classify the metagenome (the aggregate genomes of all microbes) of 300 healthy people's microbiomes across time. A sampling of five areas of the body: hair, mouth, nose, stomach, and vagina.

Why the Human Microbiome important?

The microbiome of a person can affect their susceptibility to infectious diseases and lead to chronic digestive system diseases such as Crohn's disease and irritable bowel syndrome. Many microbe collections decide how a patient responds to drug treatment. The mother's microbiota can affect her children's health.

Scientists studying the human microbiome are finding bacteria and genes that were previously unknown. Genetic studies assessing the relative abundance of different species in the human microbiome have associated specific microbe species combinations with certain aspects of human health. With a more comprehensive understanding of the diversity of microbes in the human microbiome may lead to new treatments, perhaps by adding more "healthy" bacteria, curing a bacterial infection caused by an "evil" bacterium. The HMP acts as a guide to define the micro biome's role in wellbeing, diet, immunity, and disease.

Chapter 8: Chronic Inflammation and Immune Activation

Vagus nerve can play a multi-effect anti-inflammatory effect in the system and local part of the intestine;

This effect relies on acetylcholine-mediated activation of α-7-acetylcholine receptors, which regulate intestinal barrier and inflammation through the enteric nervous system acting on cluster cells and enteroendocrine cells in various intestinal immune cells and intestinal epithelium. And flora;

 sympathetic vagal imbalance, functional enteric nerve defects and hypothalamic-pituitary-adrenal axis activity are weakened in patients with inflammatory bowel disease;

Vagus nerve regulation intervention to up-regulate the cholinergic anti-inflammatory pathway can reduce systemic and intestinal local inflammation. In small clinical studies, vagus nerve stimulation can alleviate Crohn's disease.

The enteric brain axis plays an important role in inflammatory bowel disease (IBD). A recent review by Alimentary Pharmacology and Therapeutics describes the role of the autonomic nervous system (especially the vagus nerve in the parasympathetic nerve) in regulating intestinal inflammation. The research progress of related therapies deserves the attention of professionals.

As we age, our immune system causes more inflammation and the nervous system generates stress. This is how the immune system responds to the mind. Our immune system is controlled by the vagus nerve. The vagus nerve controls the cells in our bone marrow, which can become cells in the liver, intestines, lungs, or skin. As long as we learn to cooperate with the body rather than confront it, our body is capable of self-regulation, repair, regeneration, and prosperity. "Selective" stimulation of the vagus nerve is used in some medical treatments for people with depression, or in some cases for epilepsy. Exercise our thoughts and emotions through positive exercises (such as meditation or equivalent exercises), which contribute to health and longevity. If we feel acute anxiety or stress, learning vagus nerve stimulation techniques can be very helpful.

There is an important nerve in the human body that enables the brain to make direct connections with important organs, including the stomach, lungs, heart, spleen, intestine, liver and kidneys. The vagus nerve is called the vagus nerve, and it maintains human health from disease by regulating the immune system, controlling stress levels and reducing inflammation. The body's level of stress hormones is regulated by the autonomic nervous system. When necessary, the sympathetic nervous system stimulates your central nervous system. It helps us in situations of stress, injury or infection, and helps us deal with what is considered an emergency by activating combat or escape response. When the sympathetic nervous system begins to attack, our heart rate will increase, blood pressure will increase, breathing will become faster and shallower, sweating will increase, and the area will become inflamed if injured or infected. The parasympathetic nervous system balances the sympathetic nervous system by calming and relaxing the body. It promotes rest, sleep and lethargy by slowing heart rate, slowing breathing and reducing inflammation. It prevents the immune system from over-reacting and overreacting. It is important to emphasize that the sympathetic nervous system and parasympathetic nervous system must work together and complement each other in order for your immune system to work properly. One system must balance the other to keep your body and health in harmony. If the sympathetic nervous system is not under the control of the parasympathetic nervous system and vice versa, it can lead to many types of adverse health conditions and diseases. When a part of the body is stressed, injured, or infected, the sympathetic nervous system works and triggers the body's immune system to respond immediately. The first reaction of the immune system is to inflame the compressed, injured or infected area to protect the rest of the body and start the healing process. This is often called inflammation. We usually think of inflammation as a bad thing, but if it's temporary, it's completely natural and normal. Inflammation is a sign that the body's immune system is running at a high speed, trying to protect you from more damage and make it more able to heal. During inflammation, blood vessels in the injured or infected area widen and release more immune system cells to surrounding tissues. The inflammatory process usually results in temporary redness, fever, swelling and pain. Once your immune system has resolved the stress, injury or infection, and your body is fully protected, the healing process is underway and your body can begin to relax and restore balance. This is when your parasympathetic nervous system works. Reduced or reduced stress caused by the injury or infection, the heart and breathing rate return to normal, and inflammation begins to subside. However, if the parasympathetic nervous system is not working properly, the heart and breathing rate may remain elevated, and inflammation will persist and become a chronic disease, which opens the door to health problems. Common signs of chronic inflammation may include the following symptoms (and many other symptoms not listed here): obvious signs of premature aging (wrinkles), susceptibility, acid reflux, cancer, skin conditions, arthritis, bronchitis, chronic pain, diabetes, hypertension, osteoporosis, heart disease, urinary tract infections.

Chapter 9: Dysfunctional Heart Rate

Get the right amount of exercise and the right type. Whether you exercise occasionally or not at all, before beginning every workout, it is important to speak to your primary care doctor. This is especially true when you don't see your doctor every year. Your doctor may want to conduct a physical test and may even consider performing a stress test before beginning the exercise program based on the results. It's worth it, although it might take time. The doctor can be an invaluable source of information and assistance. In addition, when you know that your doctor gave you the "all right" to start exercise, you'll have less concern.

The right amount and type of exercise is important to you. If you walk, ride and lift weights–it matters less than what you do, as long as you do it consistently. And finding a training schedule you like is crucial. The workout regimen you choose is crucial too, without being so hard and uncomfortable you are hesitant to do that, to provide you with all the benefits you need. In other words, the best level of exercise is important to find.

The extent of activity, ranging from light to moderate to vigorous, influences your heart rate and your respiration. You only need mild aerobic exercise or a combination of gentle and aggressive exercise to lessen your depression and improve your feeling of well-being.

The talk test is an easy way to oversee the intensity of your workout. You do moderate-intensity exercise if you can speak but not sing during your training routine. You're doing an intense intensity exercise if you can just say a few words without a pause for breath. Perhaps you're not working hard enough if you don't feel overwhelmed. Try to remain at moderate intensity to get the full advantage of exercising and help with your discomfort and mood.

You can try using a heart rate monitor instead of the talk test if you are the accurate type. Heart-rate sensors are reasonably cost-effective tools that provide you with immediate feedback on your workout frequency. Your age-adjusted heart rate measures the strength of your workout. For example, medium-intensity workout is between 64% and 76% and vigorous exercise is between 77% and93% of the age-adjusted maximal heart rate. You would work on keeping your heart rate at approximately 115 beats per minute when you are 41 years old and you wish to stay in the lower part of the moderate-intensity range. Your heart rate is your goal.

Chapter 10: Dysfunctional Liver Function

It may develop as a chronic subclinical and cellular disturbance. Also can go on to be life-threatening, also said to be a hepatic failure with more organ system compromise. The vagus nerve plays a series of vital roles in the digestive system, helping to control the continuing process of food descending from the mouth, passing the epiglottis, entering the esophagus, passing the esophageal sphincter, entering the stomach where the vagus nerve ensures food is prepared for assimilation and pushed forward into the small intestine, where assimilation actually occurs. It further ensures the food continues to be digested as it continues into the large intestine and the traverse portion of the colon. Vagal fibers also extend into the liver and pancreas.

As it descends, the vagus nerve reaches and influences all components of the digestive system. Together these connections form the esophageal plexus. In this series of connections, the vagus nerve plays a diversity of roles in controlling the digestive process. One notable effect is the mediation of peristalsis, the automatic contractions and expansions that move food from the stomach into the small intestine. When this process is malfunctioning, it can lead to a condition called gastroparesis, in which the contractions fail to move food through the stomach, causing loss of appetite, pain, nausea, and malnutrition.

The vagus nerve plays a critical health maintenance role in the gastroesophageal system by preventing acid reflux, which can lead to gastroesophageal reflux disease (GERD). It facilitates blocking gastric hydrochloric acid (HCL) from entering the esophagus by managing the pressure of the esophageal sphincter (which closes the opening at the top of the stomach).

Chapter 11: Chronic Stress

When we find ourselves stuck in a stressful situation, we ultimately end up activating our sympathetic nervous systems which gives us our fight or flight mode. If the stressful situation doesn't get sorted quickly and we are stuck in that tense moment, we are then unable to turn off the responses that are triggering that mode. This in turn causes many destructive problems to our systems and can lead up to our bodies shutting down. Our brains then trigger to activate two pathways, namely the hypothalamus pituitary adrenal axis as well as the brain intestine axis.

When we are stressed and suffering with anxiety in certain situations, the brain will respond by increasing the production of your hormone levels within the pituitary gland, where the ACTH hormone gets released into your system through the bloodstream.

This hormone will then travel to your adrenal glands where adrenaline and cortisol will be stimulated. These two hormones will then play a role in being inflammatory precursors as well as immune system suppressors, which explains why we end up feeling sick and worn down when we are stressed and anxious over something. We end up getting incredibly sick easily as our immune systems are down for that time and ultimately we can then slip into a depression which has also been linked to an inflammatory brain response.

We have also found that when you are anxious and chronically stressed, your brain will often have an increase in a neurotransmitter called glutamate, and when it is overstimulated and produces in excess, it can be a leading cause in depression, anxiety, and cause severe migraines.

These stressors that cause a higher level of cortisol in the system can also be a leading factor in memory loss as well as the formation of new memories. When the vagus nerve is involved, or if the vagus nerve gets damaged in any way, it can lead to unwanted symptoms such as difficulty breathing and heart arrhythmia, which often causes fainting spells, dizziness, gastrointestinal problems, and over-emotional responses.

When the vagus nerve has no control over the relaxation signal, the sympathetic nervous system stays active and causes the sufferer to have impulsive responses toward anxiety and depression.

Interestingly, a study that was developed at the University of Miami discovered that when a woman is pregnant, her vagal tone gets transmitted to her unborn baby.

This means that women who go through a stressful pregnancy, or suffer from anxiety, anger, and depression during their pregnancy will transmit those feelings into their unborn child. These women who were in the study were found to have a much lower vagal response to certain stimuli, and their children also had the same or similar response with a lowered vagal tone as well as having lower levels of serotonin and dopamine in their bloodstream.

It has therefore been found that adding vagus nerve stimulation on top of medication for the treatment of depression can ultimately improve a person's quality of life in the long run, especially for those who suffer with severe chronic depression that medication alone may not be helping with.

The National Institute of Mental Health has come to find that over tens of millions of people have gone into a state of major depression during the last year alone in the United States of America, and most of these people have reported that their depression did in fact take a hit on their quality of life overall.

Sometimes the therapies offered for depression just don't quite cut it. Even after making lifestyle changes, being on several medications, and going to counselling,people are finding that they are still not getting any improvement on their quality of life.

Neurostimulation these days is becoming far more popular and fast acting, especially for those with treatment-resistant depression. One of the best forms of neurostimulation is vagus nerve stimulation.

A study was done where a team had decided to examine the effects of vagus nerve stimulation on hundreds of people who had treatment-resistant depression. All those who participated in the study had tried at least four antidepressants and had absolutely no success with any of them before trying the vagus nerve stimulation study. Half of the participants were treated with vagus nerve stimulation on top of their current treatments, while the other half just continued their usual medication and psychotherapy treatments with no vagus nerve stimulation.

In order to truly evaluate the participants' overall quality of life, the team used certain parameters in order to get the most accurate results such as:

- The test subject's perceived physical health

- The ability to work, especially under pressure

- The ability to get around, long and short distance

- The test subject's mood at the time of trial

- The test subject's relationships with their family members

- What each test subject enjoyed doing for fun and leisure

The patients who were fitted with vagus nerve stimulators were found to be feeling much better than they had in a long time, with some improving so drastically that they felt little to no depression by the end of the study.

The vagus nerve stimulator has been shown to not only improve a person's ability to focus, but has also been shown to improve alertness and reduce anxiety in the person using it.

When a person feels like they have more focusing ability and they are more alert and active, their stress levels decline and a better quality of life can resume from there. In adding the stimulator to a patient's current medication, it can make a world of difference in that person's everyday life and how they function in society.

Chapter 12: Dysfunctional sleep and circadian rhythm

INSOMNIA

You've probably heard this term several times with colleagues or friends that are having trouble sleeping. You might have even passed it off as them being too anxious or excited to place themselves in a state of rest.

What most people don't know about Insomnia is that is a debilitating condition that has serious repercussions on the body. It is not a phase nor is it a slight sickness that sleeping pills will cure all the time.

Definition

At the core, insomnia is a condition wherein someone has difficulty falling asleep and maintaining sleep.

You, as an adult, might have experienced this a few times in the past, especially during stressful times or before a big planned event in your life. These short, phased and finite periods of sleeplessness characterizes acute insomnia.

On the other hand, there are those who have been suffering from this condition over extended periods of time. This could be because of traumatic events or biological reasons. This is known as chronic insomnia.

Whether it's acute or chronic, one thing is always constant: your body doesn't get enough rest when you suffer from insomnia. It affects your day, mood and performance.

It was mentioned in the earlier lessons that you need quality sleep. This is represented by completing a full REM cycle in which your body paralyzes itself to prevent you from acting out in your sleep.

During insomnia, people are unable to reach this stage as they have difficulty maintaining their sleep cycles or completely fail to fall asleep in general.

In today's hectic lifestyle, Insomnia has been considered as the most common sleeping disorder in the United States. More than 25 million people suffer from either acute or chronic insomnia.

Symptoms

It's difficult to tell if you have insomnia because the symptoms could easily be passed off as being tired or stressed or just the simple cause of the daily grind. With that being said, it's important to notice a pattern in these signs.

- Inability to fall asleep. Despite having the chance to lie down to get some rest, you can't seem to coerce your body into thinking that it is time to recuperate. You could either be worried about something or you feel that you still have something to do.

- Interrupted sleep. After successfully entering your first few non-REM cycles of sleep, you tend to wake up, feeling tired and irritated at the lack of rest. Even without external stimuli or disturbances, you manage to wake yourself before you arrive at your REM cycles.

- Waking up unnecessarily early. This is when you can no longer go back to sleep once you end your current cycle. You feel that you have to get started with the day despite not having enough rest.

- Errors in memorization and focus. Because of the lack of rest, you find it hard to place your mind at the right frequency needed for the work ahead of you. You also have problems remembering tasks, things and even people.

- Irritability and depression. Because of your inability to sleep well, your mood alters drastically. Since you're mostly tired by the lack of recovering sleep, you feel miserable and irritable, affecting your relationships with other people.

Besides these, there could be other symptoms connected to insomnia. You could be making a lot of mistakes at work or even worse, committing accidents while you're out and about.

The problem with undiagnosed cases of insomnia is that people tend to disregard these symptoms and just assume that they will disappear the moment that they're able to go home and get some more sleep.

This is how acute insomnia becomes chronic. Without any medical or therapeutic intervention, these symptoms just end up prolonging your suffering.

Treatment

The first step to treating insomnia is to accept that there is a pattern of sleeplessness in your daily routine. You have to stop assuming that it will all go away if you had a whole night to yourself or when the weekend sets in.

When you've recognized this pattern, don't try to solve the problem on your own. Mention it to your physician and ask for advice. Should they be knowledgeable with sleeping disorders, they may be able to make some recommendations.

This is important because you're only halfway there. Now that you know there is a problem, the next step is to finding the cause of the problem. It could be simple anxiety or something much worse. Knowing what causes insomnia allows doctors to make the right recommendations.

- Medical Problems. You might already be suffering from something else, which makes you unable to sleep. Interestingly, several other sicknesses entail insomnia as one of their symptoms. Examples of these are kidney disorders, Parkinson's disease, asthma and even cancer. You may need to go through medical examinations to find what's ailing your sleep patterns.

- Depression, anxiety and stress. These are the most common causes of insomnia, especially in chronic cases. Most people are worried about a number of things, or they could be emotionally scarred from a traumatic event from a long time. They could also be suffering from chronic stress which causes your body to feel like it is under threat despite already lying down on your bed.

- Medication. You could already be trying to solve another problem with your body by taking medicine. Your doctor will almost always ask and check your records if they've prescribed you anything that will cause you to lose sleep. It's also a good idea to take a look at your vitamins and supplements and ask about them. In other rare cases, even birth control pills have been found to cause insomnia in some women.

- Other sleep problems. At the core, insomnia could be a symptom or a disorder in itself. Sometimes, it also means you have other sleeping problems that require additional attention. You could be suffering from sleep apnea or jet-lag or even a deviation from your circadian rhythm.

Once you zero in on the cause, it's a matter of applying various methods to coax your body into relaxing. Just like the causes of insomnia, treatments can also vary.

Acupuncture for Insomnia

Surprisingly, there is now direct scientific evidence linking acupuncture to sleep problems. Studies done in 2004 have shown that acupuncture has directly caused better nights for people who suffered from insomnia.

Based on the studies, a control group that was subjected to individual sessions of acupuncture were shown to have more levels of melatonin during sleep. This, in turn, led to longer periods of undisturbed sleep. You will know melatonin as a hormone that is closely related to your sleeping and waking cycles. When it is present in the system, it prepares the body for a period of resting and recuperation.

But you can't just start sticking needles into yourself. This is an old art but it is one that requires an expert. Fortunately, there are many services that have online portals that allow you to book a session or give you access to their facilities and staff.

In case you're still in the dark about this, acupuncture is the therapeutic process of sticking long, thin needles in various parts of the body. This may sound painful and unusual at first, but these sessions have been claimed to be pain-free.

Based on ancient Chinese medical beliefs, acupuncture was initially meant to cure disease by targeting specific acupressure points in the body with needles. This, in turn, would release internal energy in the body and allow good energy to flow in through the right channels.

This system has changed over the years but is still being practiced by many experts in the field.

It is important to remember that acupuncture still remains as a complementary method to tried and proven methods. This isn't a cure in itself, and should always be taken under the supervision of a doctor.

JET LAG

What is just considered as a side-effect of flying through different time zones could be something that drastically affects the quality of your sleep.

Jet lag is a condition wherein you cannot sleep well and experience other discomforts when you pass through several time zones. Frequent flyers talk about this condition when they make several breaks through different continents, each with their own time zones.

People who suffer from jet lag usually find it hard to sleep or become really sleepy at inappropriate times of the country in which they've arrived. Because of the different time zones, you could still be greeted by the morning sun after a twelve-hour flight that took off in the early morning.

When your body expects it to be night time with the absence of sunlight but is greeted hours later by the same sunlight despite a long amount of time passing, then it's bound to cause an imbalance within your natural rhythm. This could lead to the following things:

- Irritability

- Fatigue

- Loss of Focus

- Lethargy

- Headaches

- Digestive problems

- Insomnia

Should you experience these symptoms after a long flight, that means your body is reeling from the effects of the changing zones. This means you need to get quality sleep in order to reset your functions.

Treatment

For most cases, jet lag serves as a temporary drawback to the wonders of travel. Give yourself a day of rest and your body will have completely adjusted to the new time zone.

With that being said, there are a few more remedies available to help you better adapt to this phenomenon:

- If you're staying in a new country for several days, give yourself a few days of rest, equal to the number of time zones you'll be crossing. If you're only staying abroad for a short while, try to maintain your original sleep schedule and put up with the initial discomforts of your destination. It's better than adjusting once more when you come back home.

- Adapt to your Destination. If your destination is several hours ahead, train yourself to sleep the same time the people there sleep, even if you're not yet there. Use an international clock to keep track of the time differences as you adjust your sleeping patterns. You won't be shocked by jet lag as much if you've been changing your sleep schedule before your plan leaves.

- Avoid in-flight alcohol and caffeine. These substances will only either give you a rush or a down, which are both unnecessary as you pass through different time zones. These will only tarnish the quality of sleep you get while you're in-flight.

- Use Melatonin. Think of this as one of the few cases where a sleeping aid is necessary. As you approach the time zone of your destination, you need to coincide your sleep pattern with theirs. This may be difficult especially when you're going through a large time difference. Melatonin will help ease your body to sleep during irregular hours as you try to match the time zone of your destination.

- Keep yourself very hydrated. Because of the shifting nature of your biological clock, you can never tell when your body will be in a resting or active state. Whatever state that may be, you need to be sure there is plenty of water in your system. Since jet lag may cause a change in your bowel movement as well, it pays to stay well-hydrated during long trips so that you land with an intact stomach and a healthy glow.

- Use the Sun. Don't just keep those window shutters closed. You will want to get sunlight even while you're flying, especially when you're approaching your destination. If you're arriving at night, it's best to keep the shutters closed.

These methods have been used by many professionals in the aviation industry to keep themselves healthy despite their frequent passing through different time zones.

RESTLESS LEG SYNDROME

Also known as RLS, this condition strangely finds its way as a disorder that affects your sleep.

You may be wondering how something that affects your lower appendage meddles with a good night's sleep. At the very core, RLS affects the nervous system. It creates uncomfortable sensations in the leg. These sensations vary from the feeling of something crawling up your legs, pain, pins, limpness and even itchiness.

These sensations happen even if there's nothing actually happening in your legs. They're all in the mind. Imagine these sensations happening to you as you sleep. That is how RLS affects the quality and length of your rest. People that suffer from RLS wake up in the middle of night to move and scratch their legs even if there's nothing wrong with them.

Causes

Interestingly, RLS also serves as a symptom of other disorders and diseases. People that suffer from Parkinson's and Diabetes have been known to show symptoms of RLS. Kidney sicknesses and deficiencies with iron have also been known to share space with RLS.

Some antidepressants have also been known to induce RLS, especially when taken regularly. When taken despite showing symptoms of RLS, these drugs may end up worsening the symptoms; making pain more intense and what not.

Treatment

Since RLS is connected to other diseases, treating those conditions directly contribute to easing the symptoms of RLS. This takes coordination with your physician based on what's wrong with you.

If your medication is causing your discomfort, you need to check your prescriptions and ask your specialist for alternatives that don't bring the same side-effect.

There are also cases wherein RLS sets in after you stop taking a certain medication. This is your body getting used to a now-normal routine without the assistance of your medicine.

On another note, pampering your legs a little doesn't hurt your chances of avoiding RLS when you sleep. The following tips may be done at home to help with the symptoms:

- Getting a massage. Take note that RLS is a condition of the nervous system. Your brain sends signals to your legs to feel a certain way despite the absence of any stimuli. Feeding your nerves a relaxing massage is one way of curbing the tendency of feeling pain. It's hard to trick your legs into feeling pain when they're relaxed and pampered.

- Hot and Cold Packs. This choice depends on your plans for the next day. If you're aiming for a cool night's rest, a cold pack for the legs is a great way to lower your temperature for the night. If you're already suffering from leg pains before going to bed, a hot pack will help blood circulation to bring more oxygen to your lower regions.

- Relaxis. This is known as a vibrating pad. One very unique thing about RLS is that is affects the nerves of the legs without damaging the external portion of your appendage. One way to interrupt these attacks is to provide an external stimulus to the legs. Give them something to experience to overload the nerves in the legs. That's what a vibrating pad does. Your brain won't have the time to send the wrong signals to the legs if your legs are already experiencing light vibrations as you sleep.

Unfortunately, there is no one proven cure to completely get rid of RLS. The best thing that you can do is to ensure your sleep is undisturbed by the "phantom pains" brought about by such a condition.

NARCOLEPSY

If there are disorders that cause you to avoid and disrupt sleep, there are also orders that make you sleepy when you're not supposed to be. One such example is narcolepsy.

Characterized by being excessively sleepy during the day, narcolepsy plagues 1 out of 2000 people in the United States. It may sound like a rare disorder but it's one that doesn't just affects your day. It affects your nights as well.

People who suffer narcolepsy are almost devoid of active function. Despite having the right amount of sleep, they still become very lethargic during the waking hours of the day. They tend to fall asleep easily in the afternoon, despite there being no chance to sleep well. They may even fall asleep right in the middle of certain activities.

For patients with narcolepsy, their bodies can't really distinguish when it's time to be awake or resting. That line has been blurred. This is why they exhibit symptoms of sleepiness when they're supposed to be out and about.

On top of these problems when they wake, their bodies can't really recognize when it's time to rest. This causes them to wake up in the middle of night, supposedly to do something. These disruptions in their sleep and awake cycles centers on an anomaly inside your hypothalamus.

Causes

The main culprit behind narcolepsy is the absence of a certain chemical produced by the brain known as hypocretin. Think of this as the "wake up" substance in the body.

When the hypothalamus creates hypocretin, the body is lead to believe that the time for resting is over and it is time to increase brain activity, metabolic rate as well as heart rate. These things are what keeps us up in the morning after we get a good night's sleep.

For a person with narcolepsy, either their hypothalamus is damaged or is not functioning properly, causing it to fail to produce this important chemical. Without this chemical, the body has no way to knowing when it's time to kick it into high gear or to just keep things mellow and sleepy.

Treatment

Sadly, narcolepsy is similar to RLS in the sense that there hasn't been a proven cure to fully rid someone of the disorder. The delicate nature of the hypothalamus makes it hard to cure.

Despite that, there are some methods to alleviate the symptoms and to provide better energy throughout the day.

- Forcefully boost your metabolism. If your body is incapable of distinguishing awake and sleep time, you can jump start things on your own by drinking plenty of water during the day. This will force your body to kick up its processing speeds to meet the demands of your day. About 16 ounces will do the trick

- Engage in cardio workouts. What better way to tell the body that it's time to be up and about than by giving your heart a literal run for its money? Engaging in exercise that elevates heart rate is a great way to keep yourself alive and awake and enthusiastic during crucial parts of your work day.

- Avoid processed foods. Since your body has a sleeping metabolic rate, ingesting food that takes time to digest is only going to make things hard for you. You'll end up with clogged arteries and other disorders to complement your narcolepsy.

- Change your multivitamins. The good thing about vitamins is that you can change them depending on your need. You don't just need a simple boost of vitamin C everday. Sometimes, you need iron as well. Speak to your doctor about vitamins that boost your energy and keep you up when it is most needed.

- STILL stay away from caffeine. Just because you're sleepy when you're not supposed to, that doesn't mean coffee is going to work wonders for your waking hours. It still won't help. After you burn out the caffeine in your system, your body will revert to narcoleptic symptoms at a later time.

- Use the Sun. Take advantage of your body's sensitivity to sunlight. During the morning, take a quick stroll in the morning sun to give your body a wake-up call.

Take note that these steps should be taken along with a trip to your doctor. They will be prescribing you with alternative medicines to help you deal with these symptoms. They may not eliminate your narcolepsy, but they'll make your day-to-day easier to manage.

DELAYED SLEEP PHASE DISORDER

Most commonly found in teens, this disorder stems from an abnormality with your circadian rhythm. Your body's natural metabolic rate and energy levels peak and drop at inappropriate times.

For people that suffer from this, they find it impossible to sleep in the wee hours of the morning. This is much different from a "night person" that just likes staying up late. These are people that cannot go to sleep because their bodies won't let them.

This is more of a problem with the circadian cycle of a person. It is not in synch with the body, causing a great delay in the things that are supposed to happen. People who suffer from this feel sleepy and ready for bed in the morning because of these delays. When everyone needs to go to bed, they feel like their day is just about to start.

Causes

This problem could be caused by an unhealthy development of bad sleep hygiene. Getting used to unusual hours of waking and sleeping could cause your body to adjust accordingly, changing its whole circadian clock to accommodate your unusual sleeping behavior. When this adjustment has been solidified, it becomes even harder to overcome.

This is why this disorder is seen in mostly teenagers because of their natural tendencies to stay up late. Despite that, it can also happen to adults given the proper conditions. When this happens, a solidified circadian clock with wrong bearings becomes difficult to change without drastic lifestyle changes.

Treatment

One of the best methods for restoring the circadian rhythm to normal is the use of natural light. This is also known as Bright Light Therapy.

As the name implies, the method uses artificial light to coax the body into making changes it its circadian clock in order to follow a normal routine. It's also called phototherapy. Here, patients go about critical portions of the day with a device called a light box. This box emits a bright light that emulates the brightness of natural light from the outside.

With the help of a specialist, you will be subjected to this box at certain times of the day; ideally, you want these times to be regular waking hours. Since the body follow a different cycle from the norm, the light emitted by the box will serve as a strong reminder to the body to stay active.

During sleeping hours when it is time to rest, the light box is not used. When done consistently, your body will start to build a dependence on the light from the box, changing peaks and dips in your alertness levels. During times without the box, the body will get ready for sleep.

By sticking with the therapy, you can "reset" your circadian clock and restore your sleeping habits to normal.

Fortunately, bright light therapy is also used to remedy many other types of circadian clock disorders.

Chapter 13: Lack of social interaction

Positive social interactions have been shown to cause the activation of the vagus nerve, which means you need that interaction with other people. Even introverts can benefit from talking to someone else, sharing a meal, or engaging in activity that is shared with another person, or multiple people. However, these interactions must remain positive since negative interactions and relationships can actually lower vagal tone.

When interacting with someone else, there are a few ways to increase the vagal tone benefits for both of you. First, establish a meaningful, connected relationship with the other person. This will help both of you. Making eye contact and physical connection can also be beneficial. Hugs are a terrific way to stimulate the vagus nerve, thanks to both physical pressure and positive associations.

You've probably noticed that when you get a hug from someone, it just feels really good. Some people are better huggers than others, but the connection strengthens with hugs and physical contact, making it more likely that you'll continue the relationship and view it in a positive light. All of this is good for your vagal tone and should be pursued whenever possible.

In our mental state, the effects we encounter are particularly dramatic: pain, fatigue, tiredness, and anxiety. A virtual reality simulation helps to relieve pain in burn victims by 50% more than medications alone, whereas placebos work–bogus therapies–shows us that psychological factors such as perception and social interaction mitigate the effects of biotechnological changes very much like those caused by drugs. Placebo painkillers allow natural pain-relieving agents called endorphins to be released. Parkinson's patients respond with a rush of required dopamine to placebos. Breathing artificial oxygen will reduce neurotransmitter levels known as prostaglandins, inducing many of the altitude sickness symptoms.

It may sound insane to think and believe equally for drugs, but the underlying principle behind many placebo reactions is that the effects we experience are not a clear, inevitable consequence of physical injury to the body. Naturally, such damage is significant, but our perception of it is ultimately created and regulated by the brain. When we feel stressed and alone, warning signs are intensified including pain, exhaustion, and vomiting. Once we feel safe and cared (whether it is to be surrounded by friends or to be treated effectively), our symptoms are relieved.

Part 3: Activating your Vagus Nerve

Chapter 14: Measuring Vagus Nerve function

The methods that are used to evaluate cardiac parasympathetic that is (cardiovagal) activity and also its effects when it comes to both the human and animal heart models. The heart rate with the initials (HR)-based methods comprise measurements of the heart rate response to blockade of parasympathetic tone in other words muscarinic cholinergic receptors, beat-to-beat heart rate variability barring the initials (HRV) or (parasympathetic modulation), ratio of post-exercise heart rate recovery (parasympathetic reactivation), and also the reflex-mediated fluctuations in heart rate evoked by inhibition of sensory also known as (afferent) nerves. Sources or springs of the excitatory afferent contribution that increase cardiovagal activity also decrease heart rate include:

Trigeminal receptors, chemoreceptors, baroreceptors and subsections of cardiopulmonary receptors by vagal afferents. Sources or springs of inhibitory afferent contribution include the pulmonary stretch receptors and subdivisions of visceral and also somatic receptors having spinal afferents. Merits and the limitations of the numerous methods and approaches are addressed, and directions are proposed for future purposes.

Chapter 15: Exercise to activate the Vagus Nerve

You can learn how to use breathing exercises to shift your focus away from pain. The human mind handles one thing at a time. When you concentrate on your breathing pattern, the pain is not the priority. Most of us tend to stop breathing and hold our breath as we anticipate pain.

Breath-holding stimulates the reaction to fight /flight/freeze; it tends to increase discomfort, weakness, panic, and terror perception.

You can proceed as follows: take a deep inhalation (i.e., expanding your diaphragm) into your belly to the count of five, pause, and then slowly exhale through a small hole in your mouth. Most people take about 10 to 14 breaths per minute while they are at rest. To enter parasympathetic /relaxation/healing mode, lowering the pulse to 5-7 times per minute is best. Exhaling through your mouth instead of the nose makes your breathing more aware and lets you to effectively detect your breath. When you lower your breaths every minute and enter the parasympathetic mode, your muscles will relax and decrease your anxieties and worries. The delivery of oxygen to the cells of your body increases, helping to produce endorphins, the feel-good molecules of the brain. For decades, Tibetan monks have been doing' conscious meditation,' but it is not a secret. By imagining that you inhale IN love, you can enhance your experience and exhale OUT gratitude. Such ancient strategies will also strengthen your brain, battle anxiety, lower blood pressure, and heart rate and raise your immune systems — and it's safe!

'OM' Chanting

In 2011, the International Journal of Yoga published an interesting study in which' OM' chanting was correlated with 'SSS' pronunciation as well as a rest state to decide if chanting is more appealing to the vagus nerve. The study found the chanting to be more effective than either the pronunciation of 'sss' or the state of rest. Effective 'OM' chanting is linked to a sensation of vibration around the ears and throughout the body. Such a sensation is also expected to be transmitted through the auricular branch of the vagus nerve and will result in the deactivation of the limbic (HPA axis).

How can I chant?

Hold the 'OM' part of the vowel (o) for 5 seconds and proceed for the next 10 seconds into the consonant (m) part. Proceed to chant for ten minutes. Start with a deep breath and start in appreciation.

Cold Water

Physical exercise leads to increased sympathetic activation (HPA axis— combat/flight, pressure response), along with parasympathetic withdrawal (rest, sleep, regeneration, immune system), resulting in a higher heart rate (HR). Studies have found that cold water face immersion tends to be a simple and efficient way of promoting parasympathetic reactivation directly following exercise through the vagus nerve, enhancing heart rate reduction, intestinal motility, and turning on the immune system on. In a non-exercise setting, triggering the vagus nerve is also active.

Subjects remained seated in hot-water face immersion and bent their heads forward into a cold-water tub. The mask is soaked to submerge the nose, mouth, and at least two-thirds of the two cheeks. The temperature of the air was set at 10 12 ° C.

Increased Salivation

The more relaxed the mind and the greater the tension, the faster the salivation stimulus will be. You know that the Vagus Nerve has been activated, and the body is in parasympathetic mode when the mouth can produce large quantities of saliva.

Try to relax and recline in a chair to stimulate salivation and imagine a juicy lemon. Just rest your tongue in this bath as your mouth fills with saliva (if this doesn't happen, fill your mouth with a small amount of warm water and rest your tongue in this bath. Relaxing alone will stimulate saliva secretion). Relax and enjoy your arms, feet, knees, neck, back and head relaxed. Breathe this feeling profoundly and remain here as long as you can.

Chapter 16: Passive methods to activate the Vagus Nerve

The positive effects of certain forms of massage, exercise, yoga stretches and poses, and managed deep breathing are subject to considerable discussion, debate, agreement and disagreement about the real effectiveness of these activities and maneuvers. Now, there is empirical proof that at least some of the actions do have tangible results. In particular, actions that stimulate the vagus nerve are increasingly accepted as effective and are being recommended as noninvasive, drug-free solutions to physical and emotional challenges.

Given that the vagus nerve intervenes with, or passes in close proximity to parts of the face, the lungs, the gastroesophageal digestive system, the diaphragm, exercises and actions that engage these parts of the body can stimulate and tone the vagus nerve, providing a physical adjunct to thoughtful, emotional calming efforts.

Vagus nerve stimulation is and can be activated on easily through numerous methods of relaxation and breathing techniques:

•Deep and slow stomach breathing

•' OM' or Ohm Chanting

•Immersion of your face in cold water after exercise

•Submerging your tongue in your mouth filled with your saliva to activate the response of the hyper-relaxing vagal

•Gargling loudly with water

•Singing loudly

To rehearse the act of deep breathing, ensure you inhale air through the nose and then exhale out the air through the mouth. Things to remember:

•Breathe slowly

•Breathe deeply, from the stomach

•Take a longer exhale than you inhale

To live a lifestyle of anxiety and continuous brain stimulation is to lead ourselves down a route of medical conditions and symptoms connected to high stress. Such people usually deal with fatigue, poor digestion, anxiety, food sensitivities, poor sleep and foggy brain-quality. These same people are also frequently afflicted by lower Vagal Tone, which means they have reduced the power of the vagus nerve. This particular nerve wanders through the body to a lot of essential organs and imparts signals to and from the human brain relating to said organs' levels of functionality.

The performance that it imparts is considerable. In the mind itself, it can help manage mood and anxiety. In the gut, it raises acidity, gut flow/motility and the production of other stomach enzymes. Deficient stomach acid is a significant source of gut-related health issues and an under-active vagus nerve can most likely be correlated to a countless number of health issues.

In the center, it controls pulse rate variability, heart rate, as well as blood pressure.

In the pancreas, it regulates blood glucose balance as well as stomach enzymes.

In the liver, it regulates bile generation as well as cleansing via hepatic stage one and stage two conjugation.

In the gall bladder, it regulates bile release to help you decompose fat.

In the kidneys, it encourages typical features like water balance, glucose management as well as salt excretion that will help control blood pressure.

In the bladder, it controls the voiding of urine.

In the spleen, it minimizes irritation.

In the sex organs, it helps you to manage sexual pleasure and fertility, including orgasms.

In the mouth, as well as tongue, it helps you to manage the capacity to taste, as well as saliva generation via salivary gland management.

In the eyes, it triggers tear generation via the lacrimal glands.

So just how can we stimulate the vagus nerve to guarantee that it is operating well? Allow me to share nineteen methods you are able to exercise and activate your vagus nerve.

1. Cold Showers

Any acute exposure to cold is going to increase vagus nerve stimulation. Scientific studies show that when the body is exposed to cold, its flight or fight (sympathetic) inclinations decrease and its rest and digest (parasympathetic) inclinations increase, the latter of which is mediated by the vagus nerve. Methods for inducing this include submerging one's face in cold water, drinking cold fluids, or even graduating to using a cold vest or a cry helmet. Cold showers are also very accessible and extremely valuable.

2. Singing or even chanting

Upbeat singing, mantra chanting, humming and hymn singing boost heart rate variability (HRV) in different ways. Singing from the top part of the lungs causes one to work the muscles in the rear of the throat, which helps trigger the vagus nerve. The next time somebody catches you singing along to the radio while driving the car, let them know you're simply training and initiating the Vagus nerve.

3. Gargling

Gargling with a cup of water every morning helps contract the muscles in the rear of the throat. This subsequently helps to trigger the vagus nerve and stimulates the intestinal tract.

4. Yoga

Yoga is a parasympathetic activation activity that enhances digestion, function, lung capacity and blood flow. A twelve-week yoga exercise intervention demonstrated a substantially improved mood and decreased anxiety levels in the subjects, as opposed to a management group that performed basic walking exercises. This particular study demonstrated that levels of GABA, a neurotransmitter associated with anxiety and mood, were enhanced in those that performed this exercise. Lower mood, as well as greater anxiety, are related to low GABA concentrations, while a rise in these concentrations improves mood and decreases tension and worry levels. (Reference)

5. Meditation

There are two kinds of meditation that have been found to raise vagal tone – the Loving-Kindness meditation and Guided Mindfulness Meditation. These are assessed by pulse rate variability (Reference). It has also been found the chanting of Om induces the vagus nerve.

6. Deep Breathing Exercises

Deep and slow breathing stimulates the vagus nerve. The baroreceptors or even strain receptors in the neck and center, identify blood pressure and transmit the necessary signals to the brain. These particular signals in turn trigger the vagus nerve, lowering blood pressure and pulse rate. This results in a lower sympathetic fight or flight response and to a greater parasympathetic sleep and then digest effect. Slower breathing helps you boost the awareness of these receptors, thereby boosting vagal activation. Here is a crucial tip: breath gradually, getting your belly to rise and fall. This is a planned action of the diaphragm muscle. Your traps and shoulders shouldn't be moving very much at all during each breath, as these actions are managed by secondary breathing muscles. The greater the belly expands & contracts, the deeper you're breathing.

7. Laughter

It is said that laughter is the best medicine, a saying which could very well prove true as it has been found to raise heart rate variability, something which the vagus nerve controls (Reference). Laughter has additionally been discovered to be advantageous for cognitive function and also shields against heart disease. It improves beta-endorphins, nitric-oxide levels and benefits the vascular system. It's also been found that those who set up amusing scenarios show a reduced cortisol level in general.

8. Probiotics

The gut is attached to the brain and also one of the more obvious contacts is through the vagus nerve. Within the gut is an entire microbiome, populated by beneficial bacteria, standard bacteria and yeast. These micro-organisms have an immediate impact on the brain, influencing a large percent of neurotransmitters like Dopamine, GABA and serotonin. In many cases, the human body contains less good germs than it does bad bacteria, leading to terrible neurochemistry and also decreased vagal tone. Probiotics are a great alternative to help you advertise the sustain the good bacteria along with other helpful organisms, while assisting to crowd out the bad bacteria, yeast and parasites.

9. Light Exercise

Gentle exercise was found to promote gastric motility and gut flow (peristalsis), both of which are mediated by the vagus nerve. This subsequently implies that gentle, very low level working out is able to stimulate the vagus nerve (Reference).

10. Fasting

Intermittent fasting helps you to boost higher frequency pulse rate variability of animals, which happens to be a marker of vagal tone. Once you fast, part of the reduction in metabolic rate is mediated by the vagus nerve as it detects a drop in blood glucose levels along with a drop of chemical and mechanical stimulus coming from the gut (Reference).

11. Massages

Pressure massages are able to trigger the vagus nerve. These massages are utilized to help infants to gain weight via stimulation of the gut, which is mostly controlled by initiating the vagus nerve. Foot massages also can boost vagus nerve activity and minimizing the heart rate as well as blood pressure, most of that decrease the possibility of heart problems.

12. Tai Chi

Tai Chi is found to raise the heart rate variability of individuals experiencing coronary artery disease which once again is mediated by vagus nerve activation (Reference).

13. Fish Oil and other Omega-3 Fatty Acids

Fish Oils, EPA and DHA are able to boost heart rate variability along with lowering heart rate.

14. Tongue depressors

Tongue depressors stimulate the gag reflex. This reflex is comparable in effect to singing or gargling loudly, both of which are mediated by the vagus nerve.

15. Acupuncture

Standard acupuncture therapy and auricular acupuncture (of the ear) stimulates vagus nerve activity. The positive effects of acupuncture have become more widely recognized, partially because one can question nearly all people that have had the therapy and learn of its soothing effects, as well as the restful thoughts that people have following an acupuncture treatment. I know a lot of the patients of mine absolutely love it.

16. Serotonin

Happiness neurotransmitters, the mood and serotonin are able to initiate the vagus nerve through different receptors, that are mediated by 5HT1A, 5-HT3, 5-HT2, 5-HT-4 and perhaps 5 HT6 receptors. Assuming you've been discovered to be lacking in serotonin levels, 5 HTP is an excellent dietary supplement to help you boost them.

17. Tensing tummy muscles

Bearing down to create a bowel movement means the body needs to have a rest and digest state. This is the reason many individuals feel a lot more relaxed after a bowel movement. Tensing one's core muscles by executing abdominal bracing exercises make it possible to enter a rest and digest state by initiating the vagus nerve.

18. Eating in a calm state

Do not eat breakfast in a hurry, lunches at the workplace and/or dinner in front of a computer. Consuming a meal in a tense environment can have damaging and long-lasting consequences. It's crucial to eat in a peaceful environment and a state of personal calm. Remember? Choose food that is good, Chew the food properly and Chill. Pick, Chew, Chill.

19. Chewing food well

The basic act of chewing food causes the stomach to secrete acid, triggers bile generation in the liver and bile released in the gallbladder, stomach enzyme to discharge from the pancreas and gut motility that is mediated by the vagus nerve. It's essential to sequence the digestion correctly and the body will achieve this automatically If you begin the procedure correctly. You should have time to munch on the food to the stage that it's mushy and soft in the mouth before you swallow. This will establish the appropriate sequence of digestion in movement and enable the vagus nerve to do the functions of its properly. The state digestion, sleep as well as recovery are mediated by the vagus nerve. Sticking with these habits and exercises won't just allow you to feel more pleasant, it is going to allow you to see the planet in a relaxed, calm as well as a pleasant state.

Chapter 17: Healthy Habits For Stress, Anxiety And Panic Attack

Most people suffering from chronic stress, anxiety and panic disorders develop unhealthy habit, which makes them feel more anxious, less comfortable and less satisfied. For some, their unhealthy habits – small exercise, irregular sleep, running food – had been in play long before the anxiety disorder developed, and perhaps one of the reasons why they were first out of touch with anxiety. For others, their unhealthy habits started as they developed anxiety issues. You skipped the workout because you were too afraid and afraid to have a quick walk or a morning run into your day. They often eat on the run, or eat fat and sugar when they are anxious or down. they have quick foods. They slept too much because of their depression and then drank too much sugar in their rest not to start. Whether your dysfunctional patterns have come before or after your nervous problems, it is important for you to fix these unhealthy environments.

You can learn in this chapter about the important part of the management of your anxiety and the full recovery from your excessive anxiety and anxiety disorder by nutrition, exercise, and sleep. You can hear about the advantages of regular exercise, the increasing roadblocks, and recommendations for initiating and keeping an exercise routine. You will also learn to develop a plan of regular exercise and to intensify your anxiety response by some foods, including caffeine. You will know about the importance of diet in handling your ups and downs in nervous responses, along with simple tips for improving your eating skills. You'll also understand that sleep is important - something that's not always easy to get if your depression or anxiety disorder is excessiveness - and you can take simple steps to improve sleep quality and quantity.

How Regular Exercise, Good Nutrition, And Adequate Sleep Can Help

You may have problems doing the things you know may help if you are having excessive anxiety or an anxiety disorder. If you take 30 minutes to walk around the block, you can interrupt your workout exercises, because you too are upset that an important deadline is missed. You can save lunch and eat junk food at your office because in the morning you were too busy packing lunch. And what's the difference? You don't know anyway what you drank because you didn't eat attentively. You can remain exhausted as you try to fit another thing in your day, then lie awake thinking that because of tiredness and poor sleep you might no longer be your best the next day. Yet regular exercise, good nutrition, and good sleep are key elements of any scheme that can fully recover from chronic stress and anxiety disorder.

You'll better protect yourself from stress and experience fewer symptoms of too much anxiety through regular exercise. In fact, exercise can not only reduce the strength of your stress response over time, but you will also feel less nervous for some time after exercising every day. You can shield yourself from unnecessary spikes of blood sugar levels with good nutrition which can increase your depression and worsen your mood. Good nutrition also removes your depression aggravating compounds such as caffeine, which can relax the body and spirit, or even boost your health, in your diet. You will protect yourself from fluctuations in your anxious reaction and mood, if you're not well-rested, with sufficient sleep. They will also look out against the extra stress and worry that many people begin to think about and worry about the consequences of rest.

Getting And Staying In Shape

Daily exercise is good for almost everybody, but it is particularly important if you have an anxiety disorder. Several studies have shown that people with regular exercise have less effects (Stephens 1988) of anxiety and depression, and lower rates (Hassmén, Koivula and Uutela 2000). In addition, exercise seems to protect people against anxiety and mood conditions (Kessler et al. 2005). Regular exercise has another advantage. After your workout, you will feel less anxious and feel more comfortable. In other words, although it may take weeks for you to feel less nervous to do this significantly, you will not feel more anxious after the workout, and each day you get this advantage. In reality, the more you are involved, the more so are the immediate effects of exercise (Long and van Stavel 1995; Petruzzello et al. 1991).

Your willingness to do this will affect how you practice and what amount and type of exercise you choose. Here are a few tips to help you develop an exercise routine which you will not only love but also like to do on a regular basis.

Fit an exercise routine into your life instead of fitting your life into an exercise routine. They do the best practice-regularly. The best practice they make. In other words, regular people have chosen a workout routine that works for them in their lives. When you know, for example, that swimming would be good for you, but it is difficult to do a tour of the pool (the journey back and forth, the bathing, the shower). So long as you believe you "can" dive, swimming in some other way might make more sense. Maybe it's better to just walk out of the door to stretch or jog around, or you can go and get out of work by car. Of example, you can swim if you can concentrate on it, but it may be a mistake to build an exercise schedule around an unusual activity. Therefore, when you face the pressure of turning your current life into one particular practice, you can enjoy the event less.

Enjoy yourself. Regardless of how you prefer to exercise, you will have less fun some days than other days. If you go, you will one day feel like pushing a fridge down the sidewalk, and you must drive to complete the race. You will have a glorious time on other

84

days. You'll be the same size, but you'll feel lighter and faster, and you will have an incredible sense of well-being. So running is a wonderful thing –shift your arms and legs, balance, let your body do what it's meant to do minute by minute. Nevertheless, even in days where the workout schedule is not especially enjoyed, you will still enjoy the training itself; after and after exercise, you will feel less stressed. This can help you remember when you roll the cooler down the sidewalk behind you.

If you pick a kind of workout you like: tennis, running, and salsa dancing, you will enjoy exercising more. Exercise does not mean to run a mile or to swim for 50 laps before work. When it suits your skills and interests, aerobic training can be enjoyable. You can do any physical activity that your heart pumps. You might want to choose three or five things that you may want to keep your exercise healthy and fun if you never enjoyed it. Then choose when you can participate in these things on your daily schedule. Be as rational as you can. A 30-minute walk in the countryside after school, when you have to get your child to tutor or make a family dinner, can be hard for your day; shooting your child in the courtyard with hoops for 30 minutes after tutoring, but it could be good for your day before lunch.

Reward yourself. There is a great reward for the immediate benefits of running–reduced depression and more well-beings. Track your workout routine (see following log) and use this immediate advantage to recompense you, including the decline in your stress response after training. You can also track the workout routine's enjoyment. This is a signal for you to change the routines or use certain strategies in the previous section to increase your pleasure while exercising if you have too many days low fun.

Find other ways to make a difference while exercising. Take a warm shower after the exercise for a few minutes. Good job, say to yourself; believe it. Smile, after exercise; Any work is a good job. Note, after some days of exercising you will feel great, and not so big some days. Pay yourself rather than the value of the workout. Award yourself. Use the reward plan of dot-to-dot. Draw an image that is a great reward using a sheet of graph paper and draw it. Click on a picture of your new phone or on a palm tree for that weekend, for example, to make a picture from a magazine. Put the cut-out image on the paper graph and trace it slightly. Now draw a dot where the image touches a line on the paper. Whenever you exercise, darken one point and connect with the one that you just darkened to the previous darkened dot. Take a small bonus per third or fourth point you obscure; a manicure, a movie, an hour to do exactly and just what you want to. When you attach all the points, award yourself the big prize.

Develop the habit of exercising. There are major customary stuff, like "thank you" if someone does something good for you or gift you a free ride to work in the morning even when you want to go to the beach. Yet customs can also cause problems. Take into account the anxious patterns or habits in your fearful response. How useful are these customs? Developing an exercise habit will assist you in changing the harmless habits and patterns in your anxious response. A strong habit of exercise may increase the flexibility and emotional response to objects, activities, and situations of your thinking and actions. But they can be as hard to construct as they can break, as can many habits. Try to follow R four: Routine, Reward, Remind and Relax to create a practice habit.

You Are What You Eat

Each segment focuses on improving your eating habits, particularly when you are stressed or anxious, to make sure your mind and bodywork properly. Let's get started with foods that can induce a variety of distress, including anxiety and panic, when not controlled. Nonetheless, if you have any health problems, have a medical condition that requires dietary changes and think you are overweight or underweight, address your issues with your doctor and nutritionist.

You may be surprised to know that some foods and chemicals can make the stress and worry worse. Caffeine and caffeine are the two most popular drinks and drugs which you eat daily that can help you manage your anxiety. While not everyone is immune to these foods, you might know that foods such as caffeine cause physical reactions that look very like physical symptoms of anxiety or panic.

Caffeine

Caffeine is the top of the list of all the compounds in food that can intensify the nervous reaction, partially because we eat so many foods-and we like them-that we use. You will feel irritable and refreshed by caffeine, sometimes just a minute after you have consumed it. The physical symptoms associated with the rush of excessive caffeine can be anxious and panic-induced. Apparently, after eating too much caffeine for too long, most people have experienced their first panic attack. It is fascinating that even small doses of caffeine, such as chocolate bars and soda, can make some people feel nervous and raise their heart rate and panic rush.

Caffeine activates the central nervous system directly and removes nor-epinephrine neurotransmitters from your brain which triggers you to be anxious, alert or stressed. Some are quite sensitive to caffeine and only a few sips of black tea can keep them awake throughout the night. The consequences of caffeine seem to other individuals to be impermissible. You can sleep like a baby late at night and drink strong black coffee. Nevertheless, irrespective of how receptive and insensitive you are to the effects of caffeine, too much can make you feel excessively stressed or nervous, which can make you more vulnerable to panic attacks.

We are a caffeine culture and there is caffeine in many foods and drinks, not just coffee. Caffeine is found in teas, cola drinks, chocolate candy and many on - the-call products. Limit your total consumption to below 100 milligrams per day, unless you are sensitive to caffeine. There would be about 100 milligrams of one cup of drinking or percolating coffee a day. You are halfway there with one cola or a cup of tea. You may find it hard for you to omit if you love your morning cup of coffee. But you may find you calmer and sleep better, even if you just cut back on the intake. You may want to remove caffeine altogether if you can if you are susceptible to it.

It can be hard to change your habit if you love caffeine. Yet, take small steps, if you're ready to try it. You can experience symptoms of caffeine retreat-fatigue, depression, irritability and headaches-if you consume a large amount of caffeine for a longer period of time unless you slowly decrease the amount you eat. Begin by measuring your daily consumption of caffeine.

Slowly decrease your dosage over six to eight months once you have measured your daily consumption of caffeine. If you drink four cups of coffee a day, try to reduce your target to three cups every day for one month, and then two cups every day for one month. You can replace the cups with decaffeinated coffee. This is something many people prefer as they love the espresso routine and the coffee itself. You can go even faster if you are especially sensitive to changes in the intake of caffeine. For example, you can dilute each cup 25% with water, drink it one month, then dilute it with water by 50% each day, when you drink three cups of coffee every day, and so on until you achieve your goal. Please remember that people vary in their tolerance to caffeine so that the ultimate aim can differ from others.

Sugar and Hypoglycemia

Even though you can certainly eat too much sugar, glucose-a natural sugar-is a requirement of your body and brain to work efficiently. The glucose we need is largely derived from our dietary carbohydrates, such as rice, cereals, pulp, vegetables, and fruits. All carbohydrates are not the same, however. A great number of sugar molecules together form complex carbohydrates, also called starches. On the other side, one or two sugar molecules produce simple carbohydrates, like sucrose. Sucrose is a grinding white sugar, brown sugar and honey and for that purpose, in most sucrose and sweets including candies and pastries sucrose is a popular sweetening ingredient. Sucrose splits into glucose very quickly. Starches break into glucose more slowly than simple carbohydrates, releasing glucose more slowly into the bloodstream. Complex carbohydrates are more safe for you because they do not spike your blood sugar immediately, but they slowly and steadily pump glucose into your bloodstream.

Although most people tolerate large quantities of insulin to be unexpectedly released, some people are quite vulnerable to their bloodstream rise and fall. Hypoglycemia suffer from uncomfortable physical symptoms if the bloodstream contains less glucose. You can be clam and sweaty, dizzy, exhausted and pounding in your chest. You are wrong when you say these signs sound like depression. These are some of the same symptoms reported during a panic or an acute worry episode. Hypoglycemia is common and occurs in women who are pregnant, have high fever, or have liver failure, or after other food and medications have been ingested. Although most common in people with diabetes mellitus, hypoglycemia can happen in people without diabetes, typically occurring several hours after a meal or first thing in the morning, when blood glucose levels are at their lowest. When, a few hours after eating, at midnight or early morning you feel anxious and jittery, it might mean you are suffering from low blood sugar. Try a complex glucose, such as a fruit piece or a slice of bread, to see if your symptoms are gone. When you are vomiting and getting your symptoms to disappear completely, and this seems to be a trend, talk to your doctor who can prescribe a test to find out if you are hypoglycemic.

Developing Healthful Eating Habits

Nutrition and weight researchers and experts are increasingly concerned with North American eating habits. These specialists believe that unhealthy habits have dramatically increased obesity in adults and young people. In fact, maintaining a healthy weight reduces your risk of obesity, not only your cardiovascular risk.

In addition, the US Department of Agriculture and the Department of Health and Human Services of the US have developed the Dietetic Guidelines for Americans (DGA) to promote health and reduce health risk. The DGA recommends that our eating habits be organized around three important principles:

Using little restrictions, eat balanced food. Consider the 'rule of thirds' as an easy and swift guide to achieve the goal of eating balanced food with few limitations. Include 1/3 (meat or bean), 1/3 (fruit and vegetables), and 1/3 (starch or grain) carbohydrates for each meal. In fact, add other oils, fats, and salt in your diet, and also essential vitamins and minerals (e.g. vitamins A and C, iron and calcium) to your meat. Include up to 1300 milligrams of calcium daily if you are a young person because most teenagers don't have the calcium needed to grow their bodies. So try adding some dairy in all meals and snacks.

The Mediterranean diet, which included potato, fruit, nutmeg, chicken, fish, olive oil, whole grains, and red wines, was perhaps the most simple way to develop healthy eating habits. In this way, you don't focus on eating less, but on consuming more healthy foods. The Mediterranean diet is linked to lower rates of death (Alzheimer's and Parkinson's), cardiovascular disease, diabetes, and drug-related deaths and neurodegenerative diseases. Mediterranean diet has lower likelihood of depression and anxiety than a heavily cooked and fried food, refined grains, sucrose and alcohol drinks. Although the Mediterranean diet's advantages are obvious, researchers are not sure if bad mood drives people to eat unhealthier food or better food. A Mediterranean diet, however, is an excellent way to feel better, fit and maybe add more years. The Mediterranean diet is good too. It does not hurt. Talk to your doctor and nutritionist for further advice on meal planning and diet.

Balance what you do with what you eat. Eat moderate amounts and get mild physical activity every day. When you eat large meals without being physically active your diet or level of activity is out of control. Similarly, it's neither good nor safe to reduce what you eat and exercise too much.

Exercising regularly helps you to burn more calories, builds muscle too, and then more calories are consumed. In fact, even when you are not exercise, having bigger muscles brings more calories. You may notice a desire to eat more when you develop your workout habit. Watch your appetite and eat a bit of healthy food if you have a healthy and happy weight. But, if you are overweight, maybe you want to use some of the techniques you learned in this book to control those impulses.

Furthermore, you can reduce the frequency of food cravings through a balanced and diverse diet without eliminating the type of foods you want. In addition, if you start to do anything else, food cravings usually pass in 30 seconds. When you feel the urge to open the door, rise and relax, walk around the block easily and start to work on a more exciting task. Many people confuse food cravings with thirst, so drink 10 glasses of water each day (especially if you consistently exercise them), or take a glass of water instead of food if you have hunger.

Choose clever food. These days, it is not easy to choose intelligent food. TV, television, magazines, and newspapers flood us with nutritional ads, the current diet and exercise schedule, nutrition information and medical myths. Often what or who you think can be difficult to know. In fact, it can be difficult to eat healthily with an busy schedule that takes you away from home most of the day.

When you have access to healthier choices, you are more likely to make wise food choices. For instance, 218 calories are present in a brand name chocolate wafer bar. Three mozzarella sticks have a maximum of 216 calories (each with 72 calories). You can use cheese sticks that will provide you with much more protein, even if the calories are the same if you are having a treat. Take in a desk drawer, your purse or wallet, your car's glove box or your fitness bag with a bag of healthy snack. Cheesecakes, almonds, raisins and dried fruit are outstanding healthy choices that can be easily found in the desk drawer and hold well.

Essential Nutrients for Your Healing System

Until we start, it is important to quickly address the essential nutrients we mentioned previously-proteins, carbohydrates, fats and oils, vitamins, minerals, trace elements and phytochemicals and the impact on your health care system. This will give you a greater understanding of the reasoning of driving the recovery process in reality.

Protein and Your Healing System

Protein contains the structural elements of body tissue growth and recovery and is one of the key nutrients of your healing process. Protein is the primary building block for your muscles which is the biggest and most dynamic, energy-dependent structure of your body at 40 percent of normal body weight. In contrast to its abundance in the muscle tissue, creatine is present in almost all of the body's cells and tissues, including the blood.

Sufficient intake of dietary protein is needed for children's growth; if it is not taken in the required amounts, muscles in children can result. But since the daily protein intake is only an ounce a day, a scarcity of protein is uncommon in western countries today. However, despite this, a pervasive fear of inadequate protein drives many of Western countries ' poor eating habits. That anxiety leads to overcrowding that can lead to obesity and can be very dangerous for your healing process.

Many people in Western countries have become dependent as convenient sources of protein on meat and animal products. Such diets are sadly heavily fatty and no fiber-free animal fats which pose an unnecessary burden on the digestive process. Understanding to add non-meat food into your daily diet is a much safer and healthier path to your healing process.

Carbohydrates and Your Healing System

Carbohydrates come from plants. Crops. Carbohydrates comprise the curing system's primary source of fuel. The old, common name for carbohydrates was starch, which we sometimes give to heavier, denser carbohydrates such as pumpkins and certain bread-making grain flours. Starch is wrongly thought to have "empty calories," but we realize this differently today. Because carbohydrates provide the highest overall return on calories for all food, marathon runners and triathletes generally eat lots of pasta and rice, which are traditionally "carbohydrates" before a big breed. You know from experience that this is the best high-performance, long-term gas for your flexible bodies.

In addition to potatoes, grains such as rice, wheat, oats, corn, barley, and millet are the world's biggest staple food crops, which have been a source of the world's largest carbohydrate-based nutrient for many years. Such products, which include "hard" carbohydrates, are the shortest, quicker and most effective fuels for your healing process. These usually have a lot of protein and are therefore extremely beneficial to your colon and heart health. Complex carbohydrate diet also provides an important source of essential vitamins, minerals, trace elements, and other nutrients such as phytochemicals. Your diet will consist of about 60 percent complex carbohydrates to improve and stabilize your healthcare system and keep it running smoothly and effectively.

Fats and Oils and Your Healing System

Fats and oils are important to your healing system's performance. In particular, they promote healthy skin and nails and contribute to the structural integrity of your body's cell membranes, which help your cure system to prevent infection. Fats and oils also promote the protection and insulation of nerve sheaths which improve the health of connections with your body. Your recovery system depends, as you know, on an active and precise communication system. Often, fats and oils pad and seal the inner organs in your body, shielding them from damage and keeping the body warm. Since fats are lighter than water and highly energized nutrients, they are also a convenient way to store fuel that can be used by your healing system if food consumption is inadequate or scarce.

For these factors, your daily diet needs a small amount of fats and oils. In contrast, fat-soluble vitamins and other minerals can only be ingested by fats and oils. For example, omega-3 fatty acids present in flaxseed oil and certain fish oils support the blood clotting process and can only be absorbed by fats and oils.

In certain fats and oils, there are definitely certain useful nutrients that have not yet been found. But since fats and oils are the most compact and concentrated sources of food energy, their over-consumption will contribute to obesity and other health problems, particularly heart disease as the western hemisphere's number one killer. Depending on your level of exercise and physical health, fat consumption should be limited to 10 percent to 25 percent of your total daily calories. For example, Dr. Ornish at San Francisco's University of California discovered that the 10 percent daily intake of fat works best to help the healing process cure heart disease.

Cholesterol is a big form of structural fat that contributes to the health and integrity of your healing process, particularly your cell membranes. Including cholesterol from your diet, your body can generate its own cholesterol from other fats and oils. Nonetheless, a diet that meets the body's minimum dietary needs produces more

94

cholesterol than required within the body and, if this takes place, extra cholesterol will obstruct arteries which clog and cause heart disease. Lowering your net intake of fat or reducing your total calories while increasing daily activity will help lower cholesterol levels and minimize blockages, open blocked arteries and increase the heart blood flow.

Vitamins and Your Healing System

Vitamins are organic substances that are important to your healing system's safe activity. They work with the different enzyme systems of your body and are critical to the success of essential, life-sustaining processes that lead to healthy and weakened tissue growth, repair and regeneration. While vitamins are usually needed to a significantly smaller degree than other basic food elements such as meat, fats and oils, and carbohydrates, a diet lacking them may compromise the working of your curative process and contribute to disease.

The needs for vitamins also change over time, differ slightly between men and women, and rise during pregnancy and lactation. Athletic exercise and healing from illness and injuries will improve the body's need for one or more vitamins. Due to the complexity, subtlety and still largely unexplored biochemical processes and routes of the body, it is certain that more vitamins than we know will be found in the future and accepted as important to our healing systems.

The best way to ensure that your healing system gets the right vitamin intake is to eat a healthy, well-rounded diet with enough whole grains, nuts, seeds, fruit, vegetables and a certain limit on fats and oils (specific vitamins necessitate fat to be absorbed). When a problem happens in a particular part of your body, you might need to add a certain nutrient to normal food supplies or rely on foods containing higher quantities of a vitamin to help your healing process.

Minerals, Trace Elements, and Your Healing System

Minerals are also good essential nutrients that help and support the healing process, as well as vitamins. They are required for tissue growth, reparation and regeneration to keep your body healthy and disease-free. Minerals come directly from the core of the earth and have unique properties. The structure and function of major enzymes, hormones, and molecules, such as hemoglobin, are transported throughout the body. As mentioned previously, almost every mineral component in the core of the earth occurs in minute amounts in the human body. Even arsenic, usually considered as a toxin, is needed by your body in trace amounts.

Trace elements are chemically related to minerals and typically in the same class of food. The distinction between minerals and trace elements is that minerals are needed in slightly higher quantities and have a little better understanding of their functions. We know that trace elements are necessary for good nutrition and health, but we do not know exactly what each of them needs and does exactly. Nonetheless, we recognize that a shortage of trace elements in your body contributes to an inability to thrive, decreased vulnerability to infection and even death. So while they are required in very small quantities, trace elements are extremely important for your heating system to function optimally.

Probiotics and Your Healing System

Probiotics are another group of compounds essential to your health and nutrition. Probiotics are formed by certain strains of bacteria that reside naturally in your intestinal tract. Such bacterial strains will support your immune process to battle infection, restore health and maintain the correct biochemical equilibrium in your body. It has been found that more than 500 different strains of bacteria live in your intestines and help break down ingested food while producing valuable metabolic byproducts which are then absorbed and carried to your various cells and tissues within your body. One of these ingredients is vitamin K, used as an important ingredient for blood clotting for the immune process. Researchers have found, for example, that eating lactobacillus bacteria, usually known as acidophilus, natural in yogurt and available in commercial preparations for milk and other products, reduces childhood diarrhea, reduces the chance of intestinal side effects while taking antibiotics and deters yeast infections in women. Probiotics can often successfully fight infections, particularly intestinal and respiratory tract infections. These can also reduce the doses needed and the possible risk of childhood vaccines. In many traditionally fermented foods, such as cheese, yogurt, vinegar, wine, tempeh, and soy sauce, probiotics are found naturally.

It is important to note that your body is a powerful machine with an incredible healing system that needs the best energy from the purest sources. Repair and repair weakened tissues require energy, and the energy you use as a diet will have a huge impact on your health and well-being process as a whole.

Recall consuming healthy and nutritious foods that are clean and natural, that are full of vitamins, minerals, trace elements, fluid, and protein. Such products include most fruits and vegetables, whole grains, nuts, soups, herbal teas, juices, and wine. These are also edible. Make sure that your diet includes adequate protein, vegetables, fats, and oils. Eat natural foods, which represent all colors in the rainbow, to get enough phytochemicals at least once a week. Take your time to cook your meals properly, feed regularly, skip unhealthy snacks and chew your food well. When you try to cure yourself of a debilitating disease or condition, reduce or eliminate the amount of flesh meat in your diet. Remove fatty and dense foods without weight. Be vigilant with the intake of alcohol and caffeine.

There are many outstanding food resources. When it comes to feeding your healthcare system, respect your individuality; keep your mind open and do not be too stringent or fanatical to follow a strict diet which has succeeded for other people but may not be right for you. Stay informed and listen to your body as you work on fulfilling their ever-changing nutritional requirements.

Strategies For Sleeping Longer And Better

Sleep - all of us need it, so you may not rest as much as you want as you have extreme depression or an anxiety disorder. You may have trouble eating or exercising, partially because you don't have to escape from your restless mind and body when you relax and turn the lights off. This is when worries and anxieties move in, which makes the night turn and jump. You can guarantee you're in for a tough night if you then start to be worried that you don't sleep or not sleep well.

Roughly 30% of adults suffer at some point in their life with sleeplessness (difficulty sleeping). When you are women or an older adult, your risk of sleeplessness is higher, and when mening and menopause start, you have a higher risk of sleeplessness in women. About 40% of insomnia patients have depression and mood disorder. You probably noticed that you feel more anxious and worried during the day as you sleep in poor condition. This pattern of depression, sleep deprivation, stress, and sleep is a dangerous process in many people with anxiety problems.

Many people get 7 to 8 hours per night of sleep, and people get the most from at least 6 hours of sleep per night. The body knows the way it wants to sleep and, in the early hours of the night, it becomes the longest and most essential sleep so that you can function properly. Nevertheless, the quantity and quality of your sleep could be influenced by different medical conditions. If you snore, have sleeping trouble or experience leg cramps or tingling (possible sleep apnea symptoms), have gastrointestinal discomfort, regular leg movements and chronic nightly pain that stops you from sleeping easily, talk to your doctor or a specialist for sleep. Visit www.sleepfoundation.org for updated information on sleep studies and related matters on the National Sleep Foundation's website to learn more about sleep.

Tips for a Better Night's Sleep

Several things can make a good night's sleep complicated for you. Many causes, such as too much caffeine or too late in the day, maybe noticeable. The quantity and quality of your sleep can affect your sleep habits too. Here are some sleep expert tips to help you get to sleep more effectively in the night.

Allow sleep to come naturally. When you are ready, you do not "go to sleep." In other words, you can't control sleep and you can't go to bed, regardless of how hard you try. Sleep automatically takes place, and the best you can do is leave. If you're afraid to sleep, it could be very tough for you to get out of the house. However, if you're ready it's the most beneficial attitude to be resting. So, what are you doing while you are waiting to sleep? Don't fight it if you can't fall asleep in 30 minutes. Get out of bed and try some relaxing tasks like yoga, reading, knitting, and painting. Go back to bed if you start to feel drowsy. Seek to do the same thing again if you're already sleeping in another 30 minutes. Nonetheless, don't make it to get sleep to come because of what you do while waiting for sleep to arrive.

Don't nap or catch up on weekends. Sleep pressure is that feeling of sleepiness during the day or close to bed: the stress to sleep. The first sign of sleep being on course is sleep pressure. Sleep stress is your buddy and nothing more than tinkering and trying to catch up on weekends interferes with sleep pressure. Bed pressure is reduced by capping and trapping, ensuring that in the afternoon you feel less pressure for bed.

Eliminate or limit caffeine consumption. Caffeine don't mix with sleep. The misuse of caffeinated drinks–like tea, caffeine, and sodas–and certain ingredients (e.g. chocolate) and medical products can make sleeping hard. Some people, however, are more susceptible than others to caffeine. You might be so fragile that even a small cup of coffee in the morning will make resting and sleeping difficult for you. Do not drink any caffeinated beverages afternoon when you have trouble with your sleep. Even in the evening, you may want to reduce or eliminate caffeine entirely. Don't use caffeine, in particular, to boost yourself if you feel tired. Then, walk around the block for five minutes. Use some exercise to shake off drowsiness rather than caffeine.

Exercise regularly. Regular exercise is one of the safest treatments for sleep. Strong workouts help muscles to relax and relax your worry. Exercise can help relieve the stresses of the day and reduce the propensity of your brain to revisit your busy day information. Aerobic exercise lasts twenty minutes or more at lunch or at the late afternoon. Even an early evening 20-minute stroll could help. Nonetheless, stop intensive activity within 3 hours of bedtime because it can over-stimulate the mind and body and make sleep impossible.

Take a hot bath before bedtime. As the body temperature decreases, sleep tends to come. The faster your temperature drops, the sooner sleep comes–everything else is the same. By bathing in a hot bath just before bedtime, you can use this to your benefit to increase the temperature of your skin. A cold shower does not normally work as well as a hot bath since the core body temperature of the water is difficult to get high enough. You know how the increase in your core body temperature can cause sleep if you have a hot tub or jacuzzi.

Set a consistent bedtime and wake time. Go to sleep every day, even on weekends, and get up at the same time. In the night, even if you are sleepy, at the normal time go out of bed and at the average moment, go to sleep. Consistencies in wake and sleep time keeps sleep pressure adequate and prevents the tending to drift later and later in the day for your sleep and wake cycles. In fact, the body and mind prefer to sleep and wake frequently, so try to honor that.

Create a quiet transition. Bedding is a natural way to wind down and warn the brain that sleep has arrived. Turn off all electronic devices one to two hours before you go to sleep because the ambient light from screens impairs the brain's ability to slow and prepare for sleep. Restrict bedroom sleep habits and involve all other' night stealers' in other parts of the household, such as television viewing, work, and telephone speaking. Rather, listen to the music, bathe in or draw from a book or magazine. Try exercises that are closed to your eyes like meditation, attention or savor. Thought about your day and holding it in your heart while savoring. Love the aroma of your lunch in the tasty green apple. Seek the sound of the ball during your tennis game that day when you have a close touch with him. Taste how good it felt when this project was finished or the sounds of the birds wandering that day. Taste is a good way to finish your day and let your body know it's time for rest. But don't make it to bed–no matter what you do–eat, listen, and meditate. It doesn't work! Do it in anticipation of sleep.

Transform your sleep environment. Another way to show your body that it is time to sleep is a comfortable sleep environment. Stay between 65 and 75 degrees Fahrenheit in your bedroom temperature. Remember, sleep arrives when our bodies start to warm, so make sure your bed is hot and comfortable. Sleep may be interrupted in a cold and stuffy house. Insert a light-resistant shade or heavy ribbons, making your room dark or wearing an eye mask. Finally, use a fan to mask your noises or use earplugs.

Good food, moderate exercise, and enough sleep will improve your physical and mental strength and allow you over time to manage your anxiety. Though it is unlikely that your overwhelming anxiety will be eliminated or your anxiety disorder healed, healthy habits will be a significant part of your recovery plan. Only minor changes in the exercise routine can minimize your anxiety symptoms ' intensity and frequency so that you can do what you previously avoided. In addition, maintaining healthy habits will help you keep track once you recover from your anxiety disorder.

Improving Your Sleep With Meditation

You will benefit from mindfulness as a complément to your daily life if you are one of the people in the world who suffer from sleep in a bad night. You're likely pursuing a very busy lifestyle, working long hours and changing schedules, have kids and a wife to care about and then you're yourself, clearly you have to meet needs too, otherwise you'd not be alive.

Life will always be complicated, and you will have to act quickly before this condition is harmed, should you notice that you struggle to maintain a proper sleep routine. Many people are happy to see the GP or a prescription supplier of prescriptions or any kind of narcotics to do the job, however, you risk getting hooked or addicted to the medications.

To function correctly in your life you should rest well, particularly if your lifestyle is hectic or if your career involves a lot of physical activity, athletics and practice. Athletes and sportspeople know the risks of poor sleep, energy is recovered during the relaxation phase and growth takes place with enough hours. It is therefore fair to say the mentally as well as physically, those who sleep little or no lack the vital development.

Meditation is the secret of recovery, a jumpy brain kills the chance of sleep as this kind of mind becomes hard to control, which often brings many to high levels of anxiety and insomnia. The contrary is not accurate if the brain is calm and the body always relaxes. The body is shaped by the thoughts generated by perceptions we form in our mind.

Control is necessary to stop any old idea from spinning around in the brain, thinking creates actions, and if these thoughts are not managed the same lack of control prevails overall activities, so when an individual becomes "out of control," the world reacts aggressive–all this is a huge price to pay because of lack of sleep. But it does not end, mental illness can be the result of long sleep periods, as was mentioned earlier where sleep seems impossible to achieve, but the ability to live in a coordinated way is lost, the most basic tasks are tackled, libido can be a matter of the past and relationships can take on the brunt of everything like you.

Meditation is a routine way of life to profit from. Meditation is a way of life. When it is sharp and on-line, the mind can achieve many things. The brain is the hub of thought and therefore it should function well for your benefit. Another strength of meditation is that it will calm certain areas of your brain that are stressed, uncomfortable, filled with too many emotions, meditating before bed each night, and awakening each morning (if you've been able to sleep at all), will break off the unseen layers of life accrued every day you live.

The fifth eye is hidden in these materials and we need the celestial eye to better understand nature. Once these layers are stripped, our understanding is strengthened, attention is given and the thought habits of the old varnish.

A calmer, focused and peaceful mind, which is appropriately comfortable, would allow a decent sleep. This makes you feel you are a new human being, you are prepared with a method that is always there, because meditation never changes the way people do, it never deceives and allows you to be, meditation is as it always has been; it is a way of life capable of improving even the wisest of minds, the strength-unique and unrivaled. Meditate and gain a new life through daily meditation and dedication.

Document a small change in your life by incorporating exercise every day and every night and then compare the variations in your attitude, find changes in your behavior, remind yourself how you feel before hitting the sack for a night's sleep and continue to talk to your experiences.

The friendship will grow in the forest, people will strengthen the business as, then, you will be less distressed and calmer and happier, able to talk rather than seem unsatisfactory because of the sometimes night you were born, because of counting sheep and gazing at the roof, the four walls, and the window.

You will refresh your perspective on life, and new thoughts will invade your space of thought, encouraging growth and development, achievement and fulfillment. Thoughts should feel they belong to you–because they do, new and interesting people are asked to join, and you can all afford to take the time to achieve this because your time management skills have been recently developed. Existence can be like the adversary when you are exhausted and energy-free, but it is we who crave our own opponents by the minds and bodies of its needs. That error is at all costs to be avoided if you are going to take advantage of your lives.

Chapter 18: The Importance Of Breathing Right

Breathing can be the most normal behavior for most people every day. You don't have to be careful about life, breathing moves on. Even though it goes unattended, you can regulate your breathing in a conscious way, which makes it quite different in your body functions.

Without getting too far into human anatomy, it is important to note that breathing occurs by using a large dome-shaped muscle, which is called diaphragm, and many small muscles called intercostal muscles between the ribs. As these muscles contract and relax, the ribcage and inner cavity may open up and compress, allowing muscle contraction and relaxation to extend or shrink in turn: either naturally or actively. Your heart continues to beat, even when you digest food, without your knowledge, and many of the muscles inside your digestive system function spontaneously. You can regulate your movements at will with the aid of your skeletal muscles.

Nevertheless, breathing can be conscious and unconscious. You can intentionally inhale, breathe deeply, and "suck only a little air in," or purposely exhale as mildly and rapidly as intensely and shallowly as you can actually. You can start immediately without a moment of hesitation unless you stop paying attention to your breathing.

You can also control other life functions by regulating the breath. Slowing your respiration will gradually increase your heart rate, and rapidly boost your respiration. In other words, you have the potential to excite yourself when you breathe steadily and quickly while breathing quicker. The capacity of your brain, metabolism, and virtually anything else will also affect your breath's speed, length, and rhythm and the differing absorption of oxygen. The oxygen you obtain from each intake depends on the body, and to a certain degree, you regulate the oxygen consumption.

In addition to your ability to control your breathing, your daily treatment practice would also benefit in many different ways from its biological and physiological importance. Breathing is an outstanding point of departure for focus. Breathing is always there, easy to observe and can quickly become your priority.

During meditation practice, breathing techniques play an important role. Many types of meditation like Zen meditation almost solely rely on the breathing and focus on the breathing, while all other forms of meditation would greatly benefit from breathing the right way.

It's obvious advantages to elicit a desirable calming reaction that you can change your heart rate and arouse or reassure yourself just by breath. Even if during certain sessions of meditation you can not regulate your body, it will obviously help to calm your mind.

Regrettably, most of you will live your life without ever taking care of your breathing, partly because you don't know how to breathe because you think breathing just happens. Yet breathing is much more than an amusing feature of the body because it can hold the key to your wellbeing and intensify your meditation practices.

Breathes have several health benefits through increased and more effective oxygen intake and improved use of your abdominal muscles, even though they are practiced by themselves. The bulk of the strategies mentioned in this book use the abdominal wall intentionally. Not only will this serve to stimulate the often sluggish muscles of your abdomen, help to develop a better and better, normal stance and relieve much of your spinal pressure, which partially induces lower back pain, but also deep muscles will function and become stronger if the abdomen is constantly drained and actively used with other often active muscles.

Breathing Techniques

You can try to alleviate symptoms and start feeling better when you feel breathless from agony. Let us take care of several things that you can do at any time of the day or draw on for yourself in long times.

1. Lengthen Your Exhale

You can not always relax yourself simply by inhaling. A deep breath is actually linked to the sympathetic nervous system that controls the reaction to fight and flight. Yet exhalation is related to the nervous parasympathetic system which inhibits the capacity of our body to calm and heal.

Too many deep breaths can cause you to be hyperventilated. The amount of oxygen-rich blood flowing into your brain decreases by hyperventilation. It is easier to respire too much when we are anxious or stressed to end up hyperventilating - even if we do the opposite thing.

Try a thorough exhale before you take a big, deep breath. Drive the oxygen out of your body and then just let your lungs inhale air for their job. First, try to exhale a little more than you breathe. Exhale for six, for example, inhale for 4 seconds. About two to five minutes to do that. It device can be used in any place, like standing, sitting or lying, which is convenient for you.

2. Abdomen Breathing

Breathing from the diaphragm (the muscle that is under your lung) can help reduce the body's breathing work. Learn how the diaphragm breathes:

Check-in

- Lie down on a floor or mattress under your head and knees with pillows for warmth. Or sit down and relax your head, neck and shoulders in a comfortable chair and bend your knees.

- You put your hand under your rib cage and your heart with one hand.

- Inhale and exhale your nose, realizing how or whether you breathe and move your stomach and chest.

- Should you separate the breath so that the air gets absorbed into your lungs? And the opposite? Could you breathe because your heart is going inside your belly?

Finally, rather than your chest, you want your stomach to move while you breathe.

Practice belly breathing

- As described above, sit or lie down.

- On the neck, place one hand and the other over the top of your abdomen.

- Breathe in your via your nose and feel your belly rise. Your chest will stay fairly still.

- Purse your lips and breathe out via the mouth. Try to push the air out at the end of the breath using your stomach muscles.

You must practice it daily to make this type of breathing automatic. Try to practice for up to 10 minutes three or four times a day. You may feel tiresome at first if you haven't used your diaphragm to breathe. However, practice will be easier.

3. Breath Focus

It can help reduce anxiety if deep breathing is focused and slow. By sitting or lying in a quiet, convenient location, you can do this technique. Then the following:

• Notice the sensation when you normally inhale and exhale. Scan your body mentally. You can feel the tension you've never felt in your body.

• Through your nose, take a deep and slow breath.

• Notice the expansion of your lower abdomen and upper body.

• Exhale in any manner that's right for you, sighing if you want.

• Take care of the rise and fall of your stomach for a few minutes.

• Pick a word during your exhalation to concentrate and vocalize. Terms such as 'security' and 'calm' can work.

• Imagine looking at the air you inhale like a soft wave over you.

• Imagine your exhalation, which takes away negative, upsetting thinking and energy.

• Bring your attention to your breath and your words softly when you get upset.

Use this method, if possible, for up to 20 minutes every day.

4. Equal Breathing

Another form of respiration deriving from ancient pranayama yoga practice is equal breath. This means that you drink the same way you breathe. A workshop and lying down stance helps you to exercise fair breathing. Regardless of your position, be sure you are comfortable.

- Close your eyes and be careful how many breaths you normally breathe.

- Then count 1-2-3-4 slowly, as you breathe in with your nose.

- Breathe out for the same count of four seconds.

- Be mindful of the sensations of fullness and absence in your body when you inhale and exhale.

When you continue to practice equal breathing, the second count can differ. Keep the inhalation and exhalation in the same way.

5. Resonant Breathing

Resonant breathing will help you relieve your fear and get you into a relaxed position, often called coherent breathing. Please try it yourself:

- Lie down and shut your eyes.

- Breathe in via your nose gently leaving the mouth closed and count for six seconds.

- Don't overfill the air with your lungs.

- Breathe out for six seconds, so that the air slowly and gently leave your body. Don't push it.

- Keep going for up to 10 minutes.

- Make sure you are still a few more minutes and focus on the feeling of your body.

6. Lion's Breath

The breath of Lion means powerful exhalation. To seek the breath of a lion:

- Get into a spot to kneel, cross your knees, and rest your legs. Sit cross-legged, if this position is not comfy.

- Pull your palms out, extend your legs and feet to your thighs.

- Through your nose, take a breath.

- Breathe out through your nose, let it say "ha."

- Open your mouth as wide as you can during exhale and stick out your tongue to your ear, as far as possible.

- Concentrate on the center of your forehead (third eye) or the nose end while you breathe.

- Calm when you inhale again, your mouth.

- Repeat up to six times, change your ankle crucible when you arrive at the stage halfway.

7. Alternate Nostril Breathing

Sit in a comfortable place to try repeating our nose breathing, stretch your spinal cord and open your chest. Place your left hand and raise your right hand. Then lie on your forehead between the eyebrows, with the top and middle fingers of your right hand. Close your nose eyes, inhale and exhale.

- Use your right thumb to shut your right nose and slowly inhale with the left nose.

- Pinch your nose between your left and right thumb and hold your breath for a second.

- Use your finger on the right ring to close and exhale your left nose and wait a moment before inhale again.

- Inhale the right nose slowly.

- Close your eyes again for a second, stop.

- Then, open and exhale on your left side and wait until you're back inhale.

• Repeat this inhalation and exhalation process up to 10 times through either nose. Up to 40 seconds should be needed for each period.

8. Guided Meditation

It uses guided meditation to relieve anxiety by breaking thinking patterns which maintain tension. Sitting or lying in a warm, quiet, relaxing and peaceful position could lead you into guided meditation. Then listen to soothing recordings and relax your body and breathe. Guided meditation videos allow you to see a calmer and less stressful reality. It can also help you to control intrusive thinking that causes anxiety.

Use one or more of these breathing techniques to see if it can relieve your symptoms when you have depression or panic attacks To order to discuss your problems and possible treatments, arrange a date with your psychiatrist if your depression continues or becomes worse. You will restore your life quality and control your depression with the right approach.

CONCLUSION

The vagus nerve is responsible for managing the heart rate through electric pulses to specialized muscle tissues, the whole heart is natural pacemakers in the right atrium, in which acetylcholine discharge delays the pulse.

This pulse is closely connected with the chest.

When you calculate the time between your individual heartbeats, after that, doctors can determine your heart rate variability or HRV.

This information can provide signs of heart and vagus nerve resilience.

If your always alert sympathetic nervous system revolves around fighting or flight reactions by pouring cortisol and adrenaline into your body, the vagus nerve directs your body to chill by releasing acetylcholine.

The tendrils of the vagus nerve extend over many bodies, acting as fiberoptic wires that provide direction to ease proteins and enzymes such as oxytocin, vasopressin, and prolactin.

Persons with a much stronger vagus response may recover much more quickly after anxiety, injury, and illness.

If you may tremble, or even get tangled in blood sight, or even grip, you are strong. In response to stress, your body over-stimulates the vagus nerve and leads to a decline in blood pressure and pulse rate.

Blood circulation is restricted to the brain during severe syncope, plus you lose consciousness.

But most of the time, you have to sit down or even lie down to decrease the signs.

Neurochirurg Kevin Tracey was the first to show that the revitalization of the vagus nerve could decrease inflammation significantly.

Results for rats were extremely successful, and the experiment of people with amazing results was repeated.

The implant growth to activate the vagus nerve via electrical implants showed a radical reduction and remission in rheumatoid arthritis, which is not known and is normally treated with poisonous prescriptions, hemorrhagic shock, and other equally important inflammatory syndromes.

An emergent area of the healthcare study known as bioelectronics could be the potential future of medicine, brought on by advances in vagal nerve stimulation to treat epilepsy and inflammation.

Using implants that supply electrical impulses in various parts of the body, researchers and doctors look forward to treating diseases with fewer medicines and less unwanted side effects.

CPSIA information can be obtained
at www.ICGtesting.com
Printed in the USA
LVHW011403200221
679518LV00007B/372